Functional and GI Motility Disorders

Frontiers of Gastrointestinal Research

Vol. 33

Series Editor

Choitsu Sakamoto Tokyo

Functional and GI Motility Disorders

Volume Editors

Eamonn M.M. Quigley Houston, Tex.

Michio Hongo Kurokawa

Shin Fukudo Sendai

17 figures, 6 in color, and 10 tables, 2014

KARGER Basel · Freiburg · Paris · London · New York · Chennai · New Delhi · Bangkok · Beijing · Shanghai · Tokyo · Kuala Lumpur · Singapore · Sydney

Frontiers of Gastrointestinal Research

Eamonn M.M. Quigley, MD, FRCP, FACP, FACG, FRCPI
Division of Gastroenterology
The Methodist Hospital
Houston, Texas 77030 (USA)

Michio Hongo, MD, PhD
Professor Emeritus, Tohoku University
Executive Director, Kurokawa General Hospital
Kurokawa, Miyagi 981-3682 (Japan)

Dr. Shin Fukudo
Department of Behavioral Medicine
Tohoku University Graduate School of Medicine
Sendai 980-8575 (Japan)

Library of Congress Cataloging-in-Publication Data

Functional and GI motility disorders / volume editors, Eamonn M.M. Quigley, Michio Hongo, Shin Fukudo.
p. ; cm. -- (Frontiers of gastrointestinal research, ISSN 0302-0665 ; vol. 33)
Includes bibliographical references and indexes.
ISBN 978-3-318-02578-1 (alk. paper : hard cover) -- ISBN 978-3-318-02579-8 (e-book)
I. Quigley, Eamonn M. M., editor of compilation. II. Hongo, Michio, editor of compilation. III. Fukudo, Shin, editor of compilation. IV. Series: Frontiers of gastrointestinal research ; v. 33. 0302-0665
[DNLM: 1. Gastrointestinal Diseases. 2. Gastrointestinal Motility. W1 FR946E v.33 2013 / WI 140]
RC802
616.3'3--dc23

2013048634

Bibliographic Indices. This publication is listed in bibliographic services, including Current Contents® and Index Medicus.

Disclaimer. The statements, opinions and data contained in this publication are solely those of the individual authors and contributors and not of the publisher and the editor(s). The appearance of advertisements in the book is not a warranty, endorsement, or approval of the products or services advertised or of their effectiveness, quality or safety. The publisher and the editor(s) disclaim responsibility for any injury to persons or property resulting from any ideas, methods, instructions or products referred to in the content or advertisements.

Drug Dosage. The authors and the publisher have exerted every effort to ensure that drug selection and dosage set forth in this text are in accord with current recommendations and practice at the time of publication. However, in view of ongoing research, changes in government regulations, and the constant flow of information relating to drug therapy and drug reactions, the reader is urged to check the package insert for each drug for any change in indications and dosage and for added warnings and precautions. This is particularly important when the recommended agent is a new and/or infrequently employed drug.

www.karger.com
Printed in Germany on acid-free and non-aging paper (ISO 9706) by Stückle Druck, Ettenheim
ISSN 0302–0665
e-ISSN 1622–3754
ISBN 978–3–318–02578–1
e-ISBN 978–3–318–02579–8

Contents

Preface

Though they represent some of the most common disorders seen in clinical practice among both children and adults, what are commonly referred to as functional gastrointestinal disorders (FGIDs) remain poorly understood and represent a considerable challenge for the clinician and the researcher alike. Disorders of gastrointestinal motility are more discrete and better defined but suffer from a paucity of effective therapeutic options. For historical reasons FGIDs and motility disorders are often bracketed together and, while dysmotility may certainly be a factor in the genesis of symptoms in a variety of FGIDs, other factors ranging from visceral sensation to autonomic dysfunction and cerebral representation of visceral events, for example, may also be operative in the FGIDs. Consequently, some have proposed a variety of other terms to encompass the FGIDs within a more pathophysiological framework, such as enteric neurosensory or visceral sensorimotor disorders. None has gained widespread acceptance as yet and, for now, the FGIDs continue as symptom-based disorders of uncertain etiology. The broader term 'neurogastroenterology' certainly encompasses most aspects of both motility and FGID's and has been widely adopted to describe the field of study that relates to these diverse entities. Why, then, is this book called '*Functional and Motility Disorders of the Gastrointestinal Tract*' and not '*Neurogastroenterology*'? The answer is a simple one and relates to the basic purpose of this volume, which is to be clinical in focus. Thus, the title and each of the chapters that comprise the book emphasizes a clinical rather than a pathophysiological approach to problems, be they functional or motility in nature or lie somewhere in between. This is not to denigrate pathophysiology but rather to facilitate access for the practicing clinician; a reader who will readily identify clinical problems be they symptom-based, such as dysphagia or difficult defecation or contextual such as the problems that arise in the intensive care unit or post-operatively. Indeed, clinically important aspects of pathophysiology are dealt with in detail in contribution such as 'Psycho-social aspects of functional gastrointestinal disorders'.

To achieve these goals we have assembled an all-star cast of internationally renowned experts in their given areas; where appropriate, diagnosis and management are dealt with in relation to a given clinical problem and general overviews of broadly relevant therapeutic approaches are also provided.

We believe that this book will be a valuable companion to the busy clinician as he or she struggles with challenging diagnostic and therapeutic issues and that it also provides a guide, for the clinical investigator, to the many questions that remain unanswered.

Eamonn M.M. Quigley, Houston, Tex.

Quigley EMM, Hongo M, Fukudo S (eds): Functional and GI Motility Disorders.
Front Gastrointest Res. Basel, Karger, 2014, vol 33, pp 1–13 (DOI: 10.1159/000356730)

Oropharyngeal Dysphagia and Swallowing Dysfunction

Daniel Sifrim[a] • Natàlia Vilardell[b] • Pere Clavé[b, c]

[a]Barts and The London School of Medicine and Dentistry, Queen Mary University of London, London, UK; [b]Unitat d'Exploracions Funcionals Digestives, Department of Surgery, Hospital de Mataró, Universitat Autònoma de Barcelona, Mataró, and [c]Centro de Investigación Biomédica en Red de Enfermedades Hepáticas y Digestivas, Instituto de Salud Carlos III, Barcelona, Spain

Abstract

Oropharyngeal dysphagia (OD) is a disorder causing difficulty to form or move the alimentary bolus safely from the mouth to the esophagus. The three main populations at risk for OD are the elderly, patients with neurological diseases, and patients with head and neck diseases. OD may cause severe complications such as malnutrition and/or dehydration, choking and tracheobronchial aspiration which results in aspiration pneumonia with high mortality rates. OD may be caused by inability to mix the bolus and position it on the tongue in the oral phase. In the pharyngeal phase, OD is caused by delayed, prolonged or uncoordinated arrangement of oropharyngeal structures from a respiratory to a digestive pathway, and/or impaired transfer of the bolus from the mouth to the esophagus with reduced bolus propulsion and/or impaired upper esophageal sphincter (UES) relaxation. The sequential diagnostic procedure for patients at risk for OD includes: (a) screening of symptoms; (b) bedside clinical assessment, and (c) instrumental diagnosis. Videofluoroscopy can assess signs of safety and efficacy of deglutition, measure the swallow response and select therapeutic strategies. The Fiberoptic endoscopic evaluation of swallowing test studies pharyngeal/laryngeal anatomy, sensitivity and movement, aspirations, secretions, and the effect of treatments. Pharyngo-UES high-resolution manometry measures pharyngeal contraction and UES relaxation, and pharyngeal impedance detects postswallow residue and determines risk of aspirations. Therapeutic strategies for the treatment of OD include behavioral treatments, such as bolus modification (volume, viscosity), postural adjustment, motor behavioral techniques, swallow maneuvers, and sensory and neurophysiologic interventions. Alternative therapeutic strategies include surgical procedures at the UES, tube feeding and percutaneous endoscopic gastrostomy. New peripheral and central neuromodulation techniques have the potential to induce plastic changes in pharyngeal motor cortical areas that can be relevant for swallowing function.

Definitions and ICD Codes

Oropharyngeal dysphagia (OD) is a disorder that provokes difficulty or inability to form or move the alimentary bolus safely from the mouth to the esophagus [1]. OD is classified as a digestive condition in the International Classification of Diseases (ICD) promoted by the World Health Organization ICD-9 (787.2) and ICD-10 (R13) [2]. Oropharyngeal aspiration is the entry of pharyngeal secretions, food, drink, or gastric contents from the oropharynx into the larynx beyond the true vocal folds and into the trachea and lower respiratory tract [3]. Aspiration pneumonia (AP) occurs when the inhaled secretions are colonized by respiratory pathogens [4]. Choking is the mechanical obstruction of air flow into the lungs and can result in asphyxia. Drooling (ICD-9-527.7) is the flow of saliva outside the mouth and can be caused by excess production, or inability to retain saliva within the mouth. OD should be differentiated from feeding disorders and associated imbalances in the normal feeding habits (ICD-9 783.3; ICD-10 R63.3). Finally, globus pharyngis is the feeling of a persistent sensation of having a 'lump in one's throat', phlegm, or some other sort of obstruction when there is none (ICD-9-CM, 306.4).

Prevalence of Oropharyngeal Dysphagia

The three main populations at risk for OD are the elderly, and patients with neurological or head and neck diseases. Although sufferers are sometimes unaware of their oropharyngeal dysfunction, OD is a highly prevalent clinical condition which may affect up to 30–40% of the population 65 years old or more. More than 16 million US and up to 30 million European older people will require specific care for OD by 2013 [5]. Prevalence of OD is higher in older patients with neurodegenerative diseases (80% in Alzheimer and 40% after stroke) and is related to age, frailty (44%) and muscular, endocrine or psychiatric diseases [6]. Prevalence of OD among independently living older persons is 16.6% in the 70–79 years group and 33% in the ≥80 years group [7]. Prevalence of OD among elderly hospitalized patients is much higher. Up to 47.4% of frail elderly patients hospitalized for acute illness will exhibit OD [8, 9]. OD affects more than 50% of older people living in nursing homes and up to 29% of them are tube fed, mainly due to severe aspirations [10].

Patients with neurological diseases are at high risk for OD. Between 65–75% of stroke patients in the acute phase suffer from OD and 35–40% in the chronic phase. OD is more prevalent in brainstem stroke, followed by bilateral and unilateral stroke. Around 70% of patients with acute traumatic brain injury suffer from OD, and 50% with chronic traumatic brain injury. Dysphagia is present in 50–80% of patients with advanced Parkinson's disease. Prevalence is 100% in patients with an advanced stage of amyotrophic lateral sclerosis, 30–40% in patients with multiple sclerosis and around 80–100% of patients with advanced stage dementia [11].

OD associated with head and neck malignancy is caused by the combination of disrupted normal anatomy secondary to mass effect, nerve involvement, soft tissue tethering, or tumor-induced pain and the sequelae of treatments. Up to 44% of patients with head and neck cancer treated with radiotherapy subsequently suffered dysphagia. Some 10–15% are treated with surgery, with half subsequently having dysphagia. The highest rates of dysphagia are found among the patients who are treated with surgery and chemo- or radiotherapy. Furthermore, these patients have an increased risk of nonfunctional pharynx or larynx.

Other head and neck conditions associated with dysphagia are trauma to the throat or larynx or posttracheal intubation, use of tracheostomy tubes, and cervical spine surgery. Congenital malformations (cleft lip, cleft palate), Zenker's diverticulum and cricopharyngeal muscle dysfunction can also cause OD. Cervical osteophytes, primarily with large lesions below the level of C3 and cervical hyperostosis (Forestier-Rotes syndrome) can produce dysphagia due to obstruction of the cervical esophagus from the mass of the osteophyte or to inflammation around osteophyte formation.

Complications

OD causes severe complications that can lead to death such as (a) malnutrition and/or dehydration, and (b) choking and tracheobronchial aspiration which results in respiratory infections and AP with high mortality rates [5].

The impact of OD on the health of older patients is as high as that of other chronic conditions such as metabolic and cardiovascular diseases or some types of cancer [12]. Independent of age and functional capacity, OD is associated with an increased risk of malnutrition and low overall quality of life (QoL) [7], and is a risk factor for malnutrition and lower respiratory tract infections in independently-living older persons [12]. OD has a major negative impact on QoL. In a European study, 41% of patients felt anxiety or panic during mealtimes, and 36% avoided eating with others because of OD [6]. Among elderly hospitalized patients, the prevalences of malnutrition, weakness, prolonged length of stay, impaired functional capacity, morbidity and 1-year mortality were all significantly increased in older patients with OD [9]. Up to 66% of older patients with OD are malnourished with severe depletion of muscular protein and intracellular water showing subclinical dehydration [12].

OD can also produce severe complications in neurological patients [13]: impaired efficacy of deglutition causes malnutrition and/or dehydration in up to 25% of stroke patients, and impaired safety of swallow increases the risk for AP (aspiration pneumonia) [13]. Up to 20% of patients with stroke suffer from early AP, and AP is one of the major causes of mortality during the first year after discharge [13]. Poor oral health, oropharyngeal bacterial colonization and an impaired immune system further increase the risk of AP among neurological and elderly patients. Studies have shown that AP is the main cause of death in Parkinson's disease, amyotrophic lateral sclerosis and several types of dementia [13]. AP is defined as pneumonia occurring in a patient with signs of overt aspiration or in a patient with OD in whom aspiration is strongly suspected [12, 14]. A recent 10-year review found a 93.5% increase in the number of hospitalized older patients diagnosed with AP, while other types of pneumonia in the elderly decreased [12]. Up to 55% of older patients (>70 years) with pneumonia presented clinical signs of OD, and these showed higher prevalences of malnutrition and comorbidities [15]. In elderly nursing home residents with OD, AP occurs in 43–50% during the first year, with a mortality of up to 45% [10]. Taken together, these results confirm that OD is a major factor for malnutrition, pneumonia, impaired QoL, and other complications including mortality. OD fulfills most criteria to be recognized as a major geriatric syndrome and represents a specific target for therapeutic interventions [12].

Pathophysiology

Oral Phase

Disturbances in the preparatory phase consist of an inability to reduce and mix the bolus and position it appropriately on the dorsum of the tongue. Muscle weakness or spasticity can result in failure to position boluses over grinding surfaces and weak grinding forces. Sensory deficits cause failure to recognize inconsistent bolus reduction or placement. CNS abnormalities can result in failure to initiate or maintain mastication. Abnormal bolus control is manifested by a failure to maintain the bolus within the oral cavity before swallow initiation resulting in spilling the bolus from the lips anterograde or into the pharynx with failure of the palatal muscle group. Swallowing apraxia results from dysfunction of the swallow pattern generator or from failure of sensory or cortical input to activate the swallow sequence at this level. Abnormal bolus transport in the oral phase is usually manifested by failure to clear the bolus from the oral cavity with a swallow, at times resulting in repetitive swallows in an attempt to clear retained bolus material.

Pharyngeal Phase

The oropharyngeal swallow response (OSR) consists of the temporal arrangement of oropharyngeal structures from a respiratory to a digestive pathway, the transfer of the bolus from the mouth to the esophagus – including bolus propulsion and upper esophageal sphincter (UES) opening (UESO) – and the recuperation of the respiratory configuration [5, 13]. Configuration of the oropharynx during swallow response is defined by opening (O) or closing (C) events occurring at the glossopalatal junction (GPJ), velopharyngeal junction, laryngeal vestibule (LV), and UES. Healthy subjects have a short swallow response (GPJO-LVO <740 ms), fast LV closure (LVC <160 ms)

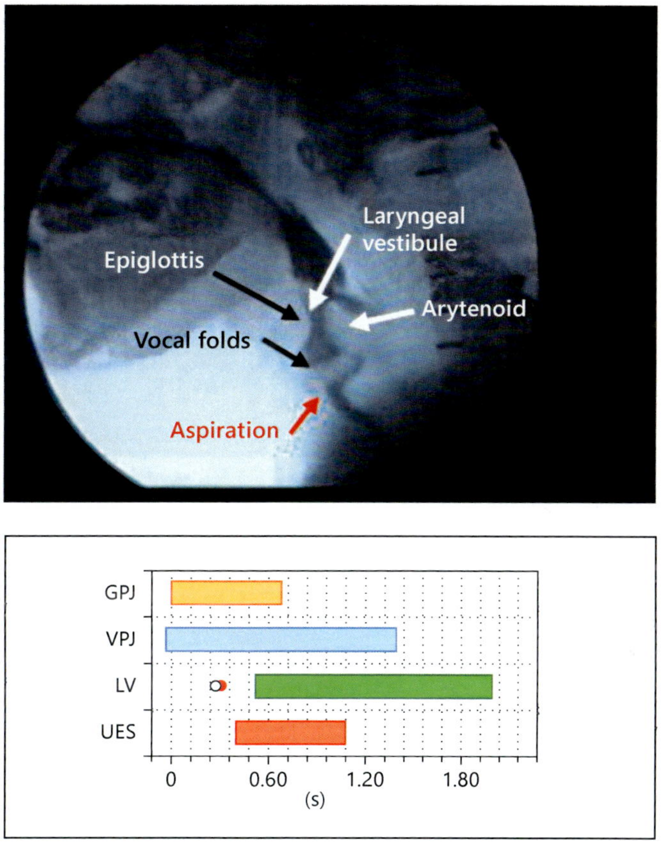

Fig. 1. Swallow response in a patient with neurogenic dysphagia and aspiration during swallow. Diagram at the bottom of each tracing depicts timing of swallow response showing severe delay in LVC and UESO. White dots represent timing of laryngeal penetration and the red point, time of aspiration.

and fast UESO (<220 ms) [8]. In contrast, prolonged intervals to LVC and UESO due to delay in the early phase of oropharyngeal reconfiguration from a respiratory to a digestive pathway are the key abnormalities of swallow response leading to unsafe deglutition and aspiration in neurological and elderly patients with OD, doubling that of healthy subjects (fig. 1) [13, 16, 17]. Time to LVC is the time interval during which the potential for penetration or aspiration occurs, and a delay in UESO increases the bolus volume held in the hypopharynx, thereby increasing the potential for bolus overflow into the LV. Reduced afferent input from oropharyngeal sensory areas, central or peripheral deafferentation, or direct brain stem damage might reduce the excitability of the central pattern generator and explain the serious delay in OSR observed in neurological patients and the elderly. Transfer of the bolus from the mouth through the pharynx to the esophagus is mainly caused by the squeezing action of the tongue against the palate providing driving forces to propel swallowed material across the UES with minimal resistance [13, 18, 19]. Pharyngeal contraction facilitates pharyngeal clearance [19]. Bolus propulsion forces can be assessed by measuring the bolus velocity prior to entering the UES. Healthy subjects presented high bolus velocity (>35 cm/s); in contrast, neurological patients showed slow bolus velocity (<22 cm/s) and weak bolus propulsion forces causing postswallow residue [8]. Older people with OD presented even more impaired tongue propulsion forces and slower bolus velocity (<10 cm/s) [9].

The Upper Esophageal Sphincter

The four main mechanisms that participate in UESO are: (1) the interruption of vagal input to the cricopharyngeal muscle allowing muscular relaxation, (2) the anterior traction on the sphincter caused by contraction of hyoid muscles, (3) the intrabolus propulsion forces caused by tongue thrust, and (4) the compliance of the sphincter allowing complete relaxation, low residual pressures and no resistance during swallowing [20]. Disordered UESO can be due to an intrinsic, restrictive sphincter disorder causing reduced sphincter compliance, as seen for example with the cricopharyngeal bar, either alone or in association with a Zenker's diverticulum. Alternatively, diminished UESO can be a manifestation of disordered pharyngeal propulsion where the intrapharyngeal forces exerted by the advancing swallowed bolus are insufficient to open the sphincter to its fullest extent. Impaired neural UES relaxation observed in spastic neurological diseases such as Parkinson's disease or brain injury is characterized by weak bolus propulsion, and reduced or even absent neuromuscular UES relaxation. A major determinant of symptoms in the context of failed UESO is the relative loss of propulsive force from the tongue and the pharyngeal constrictors. When the OSR is well preserved, extent of UESO can be normal and dysphagia mild. In cases in which the OSR is markedly weakened or absent, marked derangement of pressure-flow patterning is evident, resulting in markedly reduced or even absent UESO. The action of the tongue base is a very important compensatory mechanism that can reduce the severity of dysphagia even if the pharyngeal response is markedly deranged.

Diagnosis

The diagnostic procedure for patients at risk for OD includes 3 sequential steps: clinical screening, clinical assessment, and instrumental diagnosis.

Clinical Screening

A good screening tool should be quick, easy, and validated to identify specific symptoms of OD, such as cough during swallowing, or the sensation that something is stuck in the throat. The 10-item Eating Assessment Tool (EAT-10) is specifically designed to address the need for a rapidly administered and easily scored questionnaire. An EAT-10 score >3 is abnormal and indicates the presence of OD [21].

Clinical Assessment

The patient undergoes bedside exploration to assess signs and symptoms of OD. A recent systematic review recommends a test with oximetry using coughing, choking and voice alteration as the end points for OD [22]. The volume-viscosity swallow test (V-VST) was designed to identify clinical signs of impaired efficacy (labial seal, oral and pharyngeal residue, and piecemeal deglutition) and impaired safety of swallow (voice changes, cough and decrease in oxygen saturation ≥3%). It is an effort test that starts with nectar viscosity and increasing bolus volume, then liquid and finally pudding viscosity in a progression of increasing difficulty to protect patients from aspiration. The V-VST has a sensitivity of 88.2% and a specificity of 64.7% to detect clinical signs of impaired safety of swallow (aspiration or penetration). The V-VST combines good psychometric properties, a detailed and easy protocol designed to protect the safety of patients, and valid end points to evaluate safety and efficacy of swallowing and detect silent aspirations [17, 23]. The water swallow test (the most frequently used) has a sensitivity of 51–85% and a specificity of 66–75% to detect aspirations. However, it fails to detect silent aspirations [23].

Instrumental Explorations

If the results of the clinical assessment are positive, the patient should undergo an instrumental exploration, such as videofluoroscopy (VFS), fiberoptic endoscopic evaluation of swallowing (FEES) or pharyngoesophageal manometry to assess severity and pathophysiology of OD and the mechanisms of aspiration.

Videofluoroscopy

VFS is the gold standard to study OD. VFS is a dynamic exploration that evaluates the safety and efficacy of deglutition, characterizes the alterations of deglutition in terms of videofluoroscopic signs, allows accurate measurement of the OSR and helps to select and assess specific therapeutic strategies. The technique consists of swallowing boluses prepared with barium or a water-soluble contrast medium in different viscosities and recording a radiologically acquired video of the swallow act. Recordings are taken in the lateral and/or anterior-posterior view at 25 frames per second. VFS can be used to assess the effect of different volumes, viscosities, and food textures, the effectiveness of compensatory maneuvers, and swallow physiology in the patient. The main videofluoroscopic signs of dysphagia are: bolus penetration and aspiration, measured on the Penetration Aspiration Scale; a delayed or uncoordinated swallow response; impaired bolus formation and propulsion; ineffective swallow or oropharyngeal residue, and impaired UESO. VFS can determine whether aspiration occurs before, during or after the swallow response. Predeglutitive aspirations are caused by impaired glossopalatal seal. Aspirations during swallow are caused by a delay in triggering the pharyngeal swallow or impaired deglutitive airway protection (laryngeal elevation, epiglottic descent, and closure of vocal folds; fig. 1). Postswallow aspiration is caused by an ineffective pharyngeal clearance. Pre- and postdeglutitive aspirations occur in less than 10% of patients with neurogenic dysphagia. In contrast, up to 40% of patients with neurogenic dysphagia showed aspirations during the pharyngeal phase of swallow response, one third without cough (silent aspirations) [5].

Fiberoptic Endoscopic Evaluation of Swallowing

FEES is the assessment of swallowing and aspiration through a flexible endoscope. FEES with sensory testing also allows pharyngeal sensitivity and the laryngeal adductor reflex to be studied by delivering air pulse stimuli to the mucosa innervated by the superior laryngeal nerve. FEES can be used to study the anatomy of pharyngeal, laryngeal and esophageal structures, pharyngeal and laryngeal sensitivity and movement, aspirations and secretions, and the effect of compensatory strategies and treatments. FEES can identify several causes of aspiration which include impaired glossopalatal seal, delayed epiglottal descent and LVC, and delayed vocal fold closure, but cannot assess aspirations during swallow response. FEES can also assess the presence of secretions and residue caused by weak tongue propulsion and weak pharyngeal contraction [24].

Pharyngo-Upper Esophageal Sphincter High-Resolution Manometry

High-resolution manometry (HRM) uses a catheter that incorporates an array of solid-state pressure sensors straddling the pharynx, UES and esophageal body. Pressure measurements are displayed using a contour color plot (fig. 2). At rest, the UES high-pressure zone is a clearly identifiable manometric feature. Swallowing of a bolus produces a velopharynx, pharyngeal stripping wave, UES movement/relaxation and proximal esophageal contraction. The parameter to assess the strength of the pharyngeal contraction is the peak pharyngeal amplitude (mm Hg). Mean peak pharyngeal pressure of a normal swallow is on average 140 mm Hg, ranges from 107–194 mm Hg [25] and is known to be influenced by age, bolus variables (volume and consistency) and subject position. The extent of the UES relaxation is given by UES nadir pressure (minimum pressure during relaxation). UES nadir pressure decreases to atmospheric or even negative pressure [26]. UES relaxation duration is the time between onset and offset of the UES pressure drop. Pharyngeal intrabolus pressure (IBP) is a manometric marker for the resistance to bolus flow at the level of the UES. The IBP gradient reflects the pressure difference between UES and pharynx during transsphincteric bolus flow.

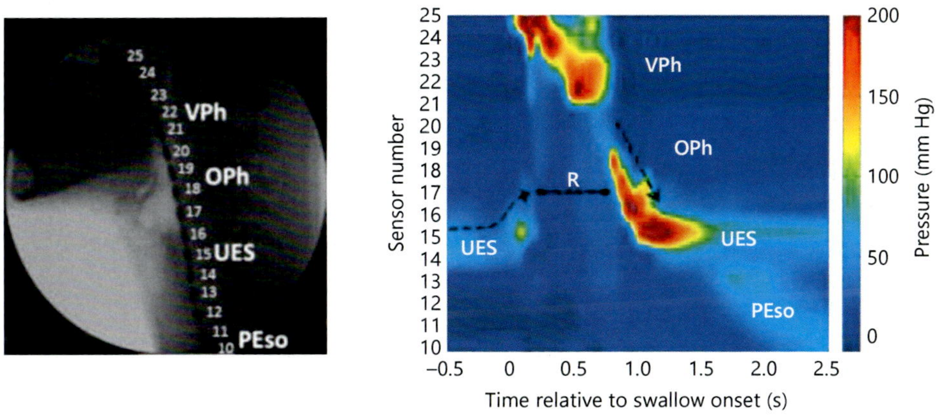

Fig. 2. Pharyngeal HRM recording. The fluoroscopy image shows the HRM catheter in situ at rest. Pressure sensors are visible in relation to the velopharynx (VPh), oropharynx (OPh), UES and proximal esophagus (PEso). The pharyngeal pressure topography plot shows pressures generated in relation to bolus swallowing. Note the proximal excursion of the UES with laryngeal elevation (curved arrow), UES relaxation (R) and pharyngeal stripping wave (diagonal arrow). Figure is courtesy of Drs. Frank Zerbib, Taher Omari and Nathalie Rommel.

Pharyngeal contraction is considered hypocontractile if the amplitude is less than 100 mm Hg. On the other hand, when the pharyngeal contraction is over 200 mm Hg, it may be considered hypercontractile [25, 27]. High pharyngeal pressures may be a compensatory mechanism masking an increased IBP in response to UES obstruction. In the case of symptoms related to a cricopharyngeal bar, manometry shows an increased IBP. A Zenker diverticulum is thought to be secondary to a poorly compliant UES unable to fully distend during UESO [28]. HRM typically shows a bolus volume increase in IBP at the time of bolus flow across the UES, normal UES resting pressure, and an adequate coordination between pharyngeal contraction and UES relaxation. Successful deglutitive UESO depends upon adequate and timed UES relaxation. A decreased relaxation interval can occur as a result of either a delayed onset of the relaxation or, a premature contraction (offset) of the UES relaxation. Both events result in a shorter UES relaxation duration but have a distinct impact on the bolus flow corresponding with these pressure alterations. Figure 3 shows an HRM of a patient with UES achalasia.

Emerging Methods

Intraluminal pharyngeal impedance provides a reliable measure of bolus presence and postswallow residual when correlated with concurrent fluoroscopy. Omari et al. [29] defined a mathematical index derived from combined impedance and pressure

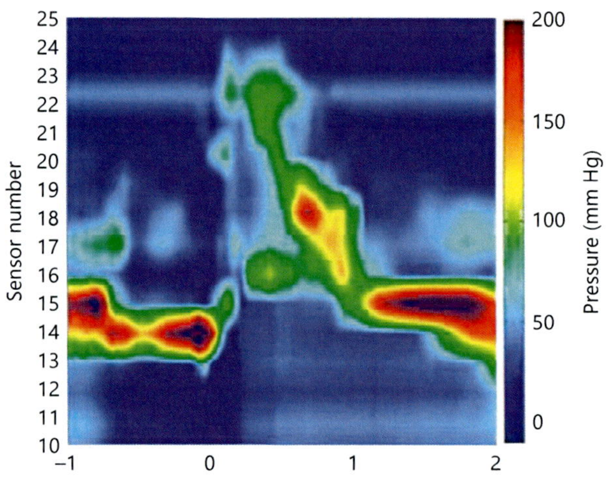

Fig. 3. Example of UES achalasia. UES relaxation is incomplete. Note increased IBP proximal to the UES high-pressure zone and below the pharyngeal peristaltic contraction. Figure is courtesy of Drs. Frank Zerbib, Taher Omari and Nathalie Rommel.

plots generated during the pharyngeal swallow. The swallow risk index (SRI) has proven to be a robust predictor of aspiration and postswallow bolus residue in adults and children with dysphagia. Whether the SRI is predictive of clinically relevant aspiration-related outcomes (e.g. pneumonia) is still not known.

Management/Treatment

Therapeutic strategies for the treatment of OD can consist of behavioral treatments, such as bolus modification and management, postural adjustment, motor behavioral techniques, swallow maneuvers, sensory and neurophysiologic interventions and adjunctive biofeedback. Alternative therapeutic strategies include surgical procedures at the UES and choices in feeding route, including tube feeding and percutaneous endoscopic gastrostomy (PEG). A combination of clinical expertise and the best available evidence-based medicine is usually needed to manage patients with OD [30, 31].

Bolus modification may include adjusting volume, temperature, acidity and/or viscosity of the bolus. Increasing bolus viscosity has been shown to improve the safety of swallowing [16]. The prevalence of penetrations and aspirations is maximal with water and thin fluids (20 mPa·s) and decreases with nectar (270 mPa·s) and pudding (3,900 mPa·s) viscosity boluses. Systematic videofluoroscopic studies found that increasing viscosity of liquids to pudding viscosity exerted a dramatic reduction in the prevalence of penetrations and aspirations [16]. According to US descriptors, liquid viscosity ranges from 1 to 50 mPa·s; nectar viscosity ranges from 51–350 mPa·s, and pudding viscosity 1,750 mPa·s and above [16]. There are also several classifications for the adaptation of solid food for patients with OD. The British Dietetic Association reviewed its recommendation in 2012 and is based on best current evidence and a consensus of experts. It should be prescribed after individual assessment of patients with OD [32]. A randomized controlled trial proved that an intervention based on diet modification and fluid thickening reduced the prevalence of episodes of pneumonia after 6 months of intervention in patients with neurogenic dysphagia [33].

Postural strategies are easy to adopt – they cause no fatigue – and allow modification of oropharyngeal and bolus path dimensions. Anterior neck flexion (chin tuck) protects the airway; posterior flexion (head extension or chin raise) facilitates gravitational pharyngeal drainage and improves oral transit velocity; head rotation (head turn maneuver) toward the paralyzed pharyngeal side directs food to the healthy side, increases pharyngeal transit efficacy, and facilitates UESO, whereas head tilt to the stronger side prior to the swallow directs the bolus down to the stronger side by utilizing the effects of gravity; deglutition in the lateral or supine decubitus postures protects against aspirating hypopharyngeal residues. The European Society for Swallowing Disorders (ESSD) recommends bolus modification with adaptation of texture of solids and fluids and postural adjustments as part of the minimal treatment protocol for patients with OD (www.myessd.org). Therapists often include oral motor exercises as part of dysphagia treatment in an effort to modify the swallow mechanism. These increase awareness of the bolus, control and direct its passage, and maximize the driving and propulsive force of the bolus in transit to the oropharynx. There are also specific swallow maneuvers the patient must be able to learn directed to compensate specific biomechanical alterations. The supraglottic and super-supraglottic swallows close the vocal folds before and during deglutition in order to protect the airway from aspiration. The effortful, forceful, or hard swallow increases the posterior motion of the tongue base during deglutition in order to improve bolus propulsion. The Mendelsohn maneuver and the Shaker exercise allow for increased extent and duration of laryngeal elevation and UESO [30]. Biofeedback provides patients with information on their physiological oropharyngeal functions using signals such as surface EMG tracings and flexible videoendoscopic or VFS images during therapy. The application of biofeedback as an adjunct to swallowing therapy may facilitate learning and speed up recovery. A recent systematic review of the literature has found statistically positive effects of these various therapies for OD [30].

In addition, these strategies can improve safety of swallow but do not change the impaired physiology of swallow biomechanics and do not promote recovery of damaged neural swallow networks in neurological patients or the elderly. However, in the last decade, new neurostimulation techniques focused on promoting cortical neuroplasticity to recover swallowing function have been developed. Two sets of strategies have been used to that end: (a) those aimed at stimulating the peripheral sensory system by chemical (capsaicin, acid), physical (tactile-thermal stimulation) or electrical (by intrapharyngeal electrical stimulation, or by transcutaneous neuromuscular electrical stimulation) stimulus, and (b) those aimed at directly stimulating the cortex, such as transcranial direct current stimulation and repetitive transcranial magnetic stimulation. These peripheral and central neuromodulation techniques have the potential to induce plastic changes in pharyngeal motor cortical areas that can be relevant for swallowing function [34].

Treatment of impaired neural UES relaxation observed in spastic neurological diseases such as Parkinson's disease or brain injury must combine treatment of neurogenic dysphagia and improvement of neuromuscular relaxation of the sphincter. Efficacy of cricopharyngeal myotomy in neurological patients with impaired swallow response is fair to poor, and injection of botulinum toxin into the sphincter could be a therapeutic alternative for these patients [20]. Impaired UESO in patients with Zenker's diverticulum or isolated cricopharyngeal dysfunction is caused by reduced sphincter compliance. Treatment of this group of patient is surgical and combines cricopharyngeal myotomy and resection of the diverticulum. Results in patients with preserved swallow response are excellent [20].

Finally, even though no absolute criteria exist, a number of dysphagia teams have deemed that a PEG is indicated in: (a) neurological patients with severe alterations of efficacy during the oral or pharyngeal stages, or with malnutrition; (b) patients with safety alterations during the pharyngeal stage that do not respond to rehabilitation, and (c) patients with significant silent aspirations, particularly in neurodegenerative conditions. For long-term nutritional support, PEG should be preferred to nasogastric tubes. For most patients requiring PEG, a small percentage of food may still be safely administered through the oral route [11].

References

1 Cook IJ, Kahrilas PJ: AGA technical review on management of oropharyngeal dysphagia. Gastroenterology 1999;116:455–478.

2 World Health Organization: International Statistical Classification of Diseases and Related Health Problems 10th Revision. 2010. http://apps.who.int/classifications/apps/icd/icd10online/?gr10.htm+r13.

3 Hammond CAS, Goldstein LB: Cough and aspiration of food and liquids due to oral-pharyngeal dysphagia – ACCP evidence-based clinical practice guidelines. Chest 2006;129:154S–168S.

4 Loeb MB, Becker M, Eady A, Walker-Dilks C: Interventions to prevent aspiration pneumonia in older adults: a systematic review. J Am Geriatr Soc 2003;51:1018–1022.

5 Rofes L, Arreola V, Almirall J, Cabré M, Campins LL, García-Peris P, Speyer R, Clavé P: Diagnosis and management of oropharyngeal dysphagia and its nutritional and respiratory complications in the elderly. Gastroenterol Res Pract 2011;2011:818979.

6 Ekberg O, Hamdy S, Woisard V, Wuttge-Hannig A, Ortega P: Social and psychological burden of dysphagia: its impact on diagnosis and treatment. Dysphagia 2002;17:139–146.

7 Serra-Prat M, Hinojosa G, López D, Juan M, Fabré E, Voss DS, Calvo M, Marta V, Ribó L, Palomera E, Arreola V, Clavé P: Prevalence of oropharyngeal dysphagia and impaired safety and efficacy of swallow in independently living older persons. J Am Geriatr Soc 2011;59:186–187.

8 Altman KW, Yu GP, Schaefer SD: Consequence of dysphagia in the hospitalized patient: impact on prognosis and hospital resources. Arch Otolaryngol Head Neck Surg 2010;136:784–789.

9 Carrion S, Arreola V, Roca M, Palomera E: Study of the body composition and nutritional status of elderly patients with oropharyngeal dysphagia. Clin Nutr 2012;7(suppl 1):172.

10 Lin LC, Wu SC, Chen HS, Wang TG, Chen MY: Prevalence of impaired swallowing in institutionalized older people in Taiwan. J Am Geriatr Soc 2002;50:1118–1123.

11 Carrión S, Verin E, Clave P, Laviano A: Complications of oropharyngeal dysphagia: malnutrition and aspiration pneumonia; in Ekberg O (ed): Dysphagia: Diagnosis and Treatment. Heidelberg, Springer, 2013, pp 575–599.

12 Cichero J, Clave P (eds): Stepping Stones to Living Well with Dysphagia. Nestlé Nutr Inst Workshop Ser. Vevey, Nestec/Basel, Karger, vol 72, 2012.
13 Rofes L, Arreola V, Romea M, Palomera E, Almirall J, Cabré M, Serra-Prat M, Clavé P: Pathophysiology of oropharyngeal dysphagia in the frail elderly. Neurogastroenterol Motil 2010;22:851–858, e230.
14 Almirall J, Rofes L, Serra-Prat M, Icart R, Palomera E, Arreola V, Clavé P: Oropharyngeal dysphagia is a risk factor for community-acquired pneumonia in the elderly. Eur Respir J 2012;41:923–928.
15 Cabre M, Serra-Prat M, Palomera E, Almirall J, Pallares R, Clavé P: Prevalence and prognostic implications of dysphagia in elderly patients with pneumonia. Age Ageing 2010;39:39–45.
16 Clavé P, de Kraa M, Arreola V, Girvent M, Farré R, Palomera E, Serra-Prat M: The effect of bolus viscosity on swallowing function in neurogenic dysphagia. Aliment Pharmacol Ther 2006;24:1385–1394.
17 Clavé P, Arreola V, Romea M, Medina L, Palomera E, Serra-Prat M: Accuracy of the volume-viscosity swallow test for clinical screening of oropharyngeal dysphagia and aspiration. Clin Nutr 2008;27:806–815.
18 Bergman H, Ferrucci L, Guralnik J, Hogan DB, Hummel S, Karunananthan S, Wolfson C: Frailty: an emerging research and clinical paradigm – issues and controversies. J Gerontol A Biol Sci Med Sci 2007;62:731–737.
19 Kahrilas PJ, Logemann JA, Lin S, Ergun GA: Pharyngeal clearance during swallowing: a combined manometric and videofluoroscopic study. Gastroenterology 1992;103:128–136.
20 Clave P: Assessment and treatment of upper oesophageal sphincter disorders, 2013. http://www.e-learning.ueg.eu/documents-view.html?eprs%5Br%5D=14870.
21 Belafsky PC, Mouadeb DA, Rees CJ, Pryor JC, Postma GN, Allen J, Leonard RJ: Validity and reliability of the Eating Assessment Tool (EAT-10). Ann Otol Rhinol Laryngol 2008;117:919–924.
22 Bours GJ, Speyer R, Lemmens J, Limburg M, de Wit R: Bedside screening tests vs videofluoroscopy or fibreoptic endoscopic evaluation of swallowing to detect dysphagia in patients with neurological disorders: systematic review. J Adv Nurs 2009;65:477–493.
23 Rofes L, Arreola V, Clave P: The volume-viscosity swallow test for clinical screening of dysphagia and aspiration; in Cichero J, Clave P (eds): Stepping Stones to Living Well with Dysphagia. Nestlé Nutr Inst Workshop Ser. Vevey, Nestec/Basel, Karger, 2012, vol 72, pp 33–42.
24 Langmore SE, Schatz K, Olson N: Endoscopic and videofluoroscopic evaluations of swallowing and aspiration. Ann Otol Rhinol Laryngol 1991;100:678–681.
25 Omari TI, Dejaeger E, van Beckevoort D, Goeleven A, Davidson GP, Dent J, Tack J, Rommel N: A method to objectively assess swallow function in adults with suspected aspiration. Gastroenterology 2011; 140:1454–1463.
26 McCulloch TM, Hoffman MR, Ciucci MR: High-resolution manometry of pharyngeal swallow pressure events associated with head turn and chin tuck. Ann Otology Rhinol Laryngol 2010;119:369–376.
27 Massey BT: Cricopharyngeal achalasia; in Shaker R (ed): Manual of Diagnostic and Therapeutic Techniques for Disorders of Deglutition. Berlin, Springer, 2013, pp 515–527.
28 Cook IJ: Zenker's diverticulum; in Shaker R (ed): Manual of Diagnostic and Therapeutic Techniques for Disorders of Deglutition. Berlin, Springer, 2013, pp 495–508.
29 Omari TI, Dejaeger E, Tack J, Van Beckevoort D, Rommel N: Effect of bolus volume and viscosity on pharyngeal automated impedance manometry variables derived for broad dysphagia patients. Dysphagia DOI: 10.1007/s00455-012-9423-z.
30 Speyer R, Baijens L, Heijnen M, Zwijnenberg I: Effects of therapy in oropharyngeal dysphagia by speech and language therapists: a systematic review. Dysphagia 2010;25:40–65.
31 Geeganage C, Beavan J, Ellender S, Bath PMW: Interventions for dysphagia and nutritional support in acute and subacute stroke. Cochrane Database Syst Rev 2012;10:CD000323.
32 The British Dietetic Association: Dysphagia Diet Food Texture Descriptors (2013). http://www.bda.uk.com/publications/statements/NationalDescriptors TextureModificationAdults.pdf.
33 Groher ME: Dysphagic patients with progressive neurologic disease. Semin Neurol 1996;16:355–363.
34 Rofes L, Vilardell N, Clavé P: Post-stroke dysphagia: progress at last. Neurogastroenterol Motil 2013;25(4):278–282.

Daniel Sifrim, MD, PhD
Barts and The London School of Medicine and Dentistry
Wingate Institute of Neurogastroenterology, 26 Ashfield Street
London E12AJ (UK)
E-Mail d.sifrim@qmul.ac.uk

Quigley EMM, Hongo M, Fukudo S (eds): Functional and GI Motility Disorders.
Front Gastrointest Res. Basel, Karger, 2014, vol 33, pp 14–24 (DOI: 10.1159/000356732)

Nonobstructive Dysphagia

Michio Hongo[a, b] · Tomotaka Shoji[c] · Yuka Endo[c]

[a]Tohoku University, Sendai, [b]Kurokawa General Hospital, Taiwa, and [c]Psychosomatic Medicine, Tohoku University Hospital, Sendai, Japan

Abstract

Nonobstructive dysphagia is a disorder where there is a sensation of food sticking in the esophagus in the absence of mechanical obstruction in the esophageal body. Symptom evaluation and exclusion of mechanical obstruction is essential for the diagnosis of nonobstructive dysphagia. Evaluation of pathophysiology of nonobstructive dysphagia is targeted at the identification of abnormal transit of the swallowed bolus using such techniques as a transit study or manometry. Classically, transit was evaluated by a barium swallow or scintigraphy. The recent development of a technology combining intraluminal multichannel impedance measurements with manometry allows the evaluation of precise correlations between the passage of the bolus and mechanical function of the esophagus. Also, manometry itself has progressed with the advent of multichannel high-resolution manometry. The interruption of peristaltic propagation in the esophagus may induce dysphagia at the transitional zone or in a diverticulum. More than a half of the patients with nonobstructive dysphagia show dysmotility of the esophagus. Ineffective esophageal motility is the most frequently found abnormality, followed by diffuse esophageal spasm. However, 40% of patients with nonobstructive dysphagia will demonstrate normal motility. Among dysphagia patients with normal motility, some may have abnormal transit. Dysphagia is a common symptom in patients with eosinophilic esophagitis (EoE). EoE patients show decreased distensibility, leading to resistance in the esophagus. Combined impedance and manometry studies in EoE show abnormal bolus transit suggesting the presence of a similar phenomenon in EoE to those with nonobstructive dysphagia. Though the majority of patients with nonobstructive dysphagia have some kind of esophageal dysmotility, its precise pathophysiology is not clear. Firm guidelines for the treatment of nonobstructive dysphagia have not been established, as yet. However, empiric dilatation to a diameter of 15–17 mm may provide good long-term efficacy. This suggests that patients with nonobstructive dysphagia may have some form of esophageal resistance, which might be responsible for the symptom of dysphagia.

Definition of Dysphagia

Dysphagia is a sensation of difficulty in swallowing. Swallowing starts at the oral cavity where deglutition is initiated, and is followed by pharyngeal deglutition. The ingested bolus passes through the pharynx and enters into the esophagus via the upper esophageal sphincter. The esophagus transports the bolus distally through its peristaltic function. During the transport of the bolus in the esophagus, the lower esophageal sphincter (LES) at the distal end of the esophagus opens to allow the passage of the bolus into the stomach. In this manner, peristaltic function of the esophageal body and relaxation of LES play key roles in the transport of the bolus through the esophagus. When the transit of the ingested bolus is interrupted, it may stick in the esophagus, leading to the symptom of dysphagia.

Dysphagia may reflect two different sensations or physical functions: (1) difficulty in deglutition, and (2) a sensation of the ingested bolus sticking in the esophagus or retrosternal area. The former sensation, difficulty in deglutition, can be defined as oropharyngeal dysphagia. The latter sensation, the ingested bolus sticking in the esophagus or retrosternal area, is defined as esophageal dysphagia. The sensation of a mass in the pharynx or upper esophageal area belongs to quite a different category and is defined as globus sensation. Odynophagia, or painful swallowing, caused by esophageal infections such as the viruses herpes simplex and cytomegalovirus, and candida, should be carefully distinguished from dysphagia.

Definition of Nonobstructive Dysphagia

Nonobstructive dysphagia is defined as a subjective symptom of dysphagia in the absence of mechanical obstruction. The symptom of dysphagia can, in turn, be described as a sensation of impaired bolus passage through the esophagus. When the symptom is triggered by dysfunction at the level of the LES, it is classified as achalasia and its related disorders. Causes of mechanical obstruction leading to the development of dysphagia include tumors arising from esophagus, peptic strictures, Schatzki rings, webs, radiation injury, and extrinsic compression by any structure outside of the esophagus. Therefore, before nonobstructive dysphagia is considered, these conditions causing esophageal narrowing should be excluded. It is not clear at this time whether eosinophilic esophagitis (EoE) should be classified as a nonobstructive cause or mechanical cause of dysphagia.

Possible Mechanism of Nonobstructive Dysphagia

Dysphagia is a symptom suggestive of impaired bolus transit in the esophagus. Possible mechanisms causing such phenomena are listed in table 1.

Table 1. Possible mechanism of impaired bolus transit

1. Abnormal motility with impaired bolus transit
   - a loss of contractile activity
   - b weak peristaltic activity
   - c impaired peristaltic sequence
     - i interrupted peristalsis
     - ii impaired peristaltic sequence (interrupted, repetitive and/or simultaneous)
2. Normal motility with impaired bolus transit
   - i deficiency in pharyngeal propulsive force
   - ii impaired esophageal accommodation/increased resistance

Table 2. Diagnostic steps in the evaluation of nonobstructive dysphagia

1. Confirm history of dysphagia
2. Exclude mechanical obstruction in the esophageal lumen
3. Evaluation of pathophysiology
   - a Bolus transit study
     - i Barium swallow
     - ii Scintigraphic study
     - iii Multi-channel intraluminal impedance study
   - b Manometry
     - i Conventional manometry
     - ii HRM

Abnormal motility most likely causes impaired bolus transit causing the symptom of dysphagia as a consequence of: (a) loss of peristaltic force of the esophagus, (b) weak peristaltic force of the esophagus, (c) impaired formation of the peristaltic sequence such as interruption in the peristaltic sequence, and interrupted peristaltic sequence due to repetitive and/or simultaneous contractions.

There are a certain proportion of patients with dysphagia with normal manometry and transit. The precise mechanism leading to the development of abnormal transit in the individual with normal manometry has not, as yet, been clarified.

Diagnosing Nonobstructive Dysphagia

For the diagnosis of nonobstructive dysphagia, symptom evaluation and exclusion of mechanical obstruction is essential. Evaluation of pathophysiology is important, but our current knowledge does not permit a complete explanation of pathophysiology in all cases (table 2).

Evaluation of Symptom

According to the definition of nonobstructive dysphagia, this condition is diagnosed by the confirmation of the symptom of dysphagia in the absence of mechanical obstruction. Conventionally, exclusion of mechanical obstruction can be made by fluoroscopic study with barium swallow or endoscopy, irrespective of the pathologic diagnosis underlying esophageal narrowing.

Though the term dysphagia includes difficulties in the oropharyngeal region and in the esophageal region, these should be separated. Oropharyngeal dysphagia can be described as difficulty in control of food in the mouth, difficulty initiating a swallow, coughing, choking or wet voice after swallowing. In oropharyngeal dysphagia, the patient may complain that the food is getting stuck in the region of the neck or suprasternal notch. Esophageal dysphagia presents as food sticking in the middle of the chest, or tightening or swelling of the throat [1]. Food impaction might be reported in some patients. Dysphagia of acute onset, which is progressive, where there is an inability to ingest food, or where regurgitation is present, may suggest mechanical obstruction. Before making a clinical diagnosis of esophageal dysphagia, the clinician should carefully examine symptoms to confirm that they suggest an esophageal and not an oropharyngeal origin.

Exclusion of Obstructive Mechanical Lesions

Endoscopy is the essential diagnostic tool to exclude mechanical obstruction of the esophageal lumen. However, external compression by advanced sclerosis of aorta or aortic aneurysm (dysphagia aortica) [2] or an aberrant right subclavian artery (dysphagia lusoria) [3] might remain undiagnosed due the esophageal distention during an endoscopic procedure. In such case, conventional barium swallow may show such subtle changes as vascular compression. If any suspicious lesion obstructing the lumen of the esophagus is identified by barium swallow or endoscopy, further extensive diagnostic studies should be applied if there is any possibility of the presence of an underlying malignancy.

Evaluation of Pathophysiology

For the evaluation of nonobstructive dysphagia, bolus transit studies and manometry may be employed [4].

Bolus Transit Study

Traditionally, transit was assessed by fluoroscopy; typically, by a video-fluoroscopic study. Barium is thc standard material used in a fluoroscopic transit study, but barium-coated marshmallow can also be used to evaluate solid bolus transit. Scintigraphic studies provide a semiquantitative evaluation of transit of either liquid or a more viscous material. The more recently introduced technology, multichannel intraluminal impedance, may provide more precise dynamics of bolus transit in the esophagus. Usually, an impedance transit study is performed with manometry to examine correlations between bolus transit and contractile activities of the esophagus.

Manometry

Manometric studies with widely spaced sensors were originally used for clinical evaluation of esophageal motor function but have been rapidly replaced by high-resolution manometry (HRM) involving closely spaced sensors, often combined with multichannel intraluminal impedance. HRM provides an assessment of esophageal contractile function along the entire length of esophagus, which enables more precise evaluation of motor function of the esophagus [5] as a pressure trough in peristaltic amplitude in the peristaltic sequence may contribute to impaired bolus transit. Such troughs, if less than 5 cm in length might go unrecognized with conventional manometry where sensors are spaced 5 cm apart. HRM uncovers such subtle findings. When combined with multichannel intraluminal impedance, relationships between passage of bolus and esophageal contractile activity can be evaluated.

Manometric Diagnosis in Patients with Nonobstructive Dysphagia

Many studies have reported on manometric diagnoses in patients with nonobstructive dysphagia. It is not appropriate to include achalasia within the category of nonobstructive dysphagia. Excluding achalasia, an esophageal motor abnormality is the major finding: ineffective esophageal motility or nonspecific esophageal motor disorders being described in 40% of patients and diffuse esophageal spasm (DES) in 20% of patients. Nutcracker esophagus can be found in 1% of patients (table 3) [6–10]. Ineffective esophageal motility features weak esophageal contractions which are not sufficient to propel the bolus through the esophagus, and, in DES, the loss of effective peristaltic sequence results in failure to transport the bolus. Though esophageal dysmotility is frequently identified among patients with nonobstructive dysphagia, 40% of patients with dysphagia show normal manometry.

Weak Peristalsis

Peristaltic integrity is critical to clearing luminal content from the esophagus [11]. In a classic study, peristaltic contractions with the amplitude >12 mm Hg in proximal esophagus and >25 mm Hg in the distal esophagus were reported as being capable of preventing retrograde escape of swallowed barium [11]. A recent study employing

Table 3. Manometric findings in patients with nonobstructive dysphagia

	Schoeman et al. [6]	Conchillo et al. [7]	Burgess et al. [8]	Nguyen et al. [9]	Chen et al. [10]	Sum	Percentage	
							total	excl. ach.
Total number of patients	30	40	41	42	18	171	171	138
Normal motility	9	20	4	11	10	54	32%	39%
IEM	10	13	5	19	8	55	32%	40%
DES	11	4	7	5	–	27	16%	20%
NCE	–	–	2	–	–	2	5%	1%
Achalasia	–	3	23	7	–	33	19%	–

Note: achalasia is included in some studies and not in others. IEM = Ineffective esophageal motility; NCE = nutcracker esophagus; Sum = sum of the number of patients studied; excl. ach. = excluding achalasia.

HRM reconfirmed that a break in the pressure profile featuring peristaltic amplitudes of less than 20 mm Hg resulted in incomplete bolus transit [12]. In manometric studies in nonobstructive dysphagia, ineffective esophageal manometry is the most frequently found abnormality (table 3).

Impaired Peristalsis

Manometric studies in nonobstructive dysphagia patients also show a high prevalence of conditions such as DES (20%).

Interruption of Peristalsis

Though not included in many series reporting on nonobstructive dysphagia, the interruption of the peristaltic pressure sequence is now recognized as an important mechanism causing impaired transit associated with abnormal motility. It has been well known that the transitional zone between the striated and smooth muscle portions of the esophagus is associated with a trough in the manometric profile of the esophagus, but, usually, such a minor pressure trough does not induce the symptom of dysphagia. HRM revealed a second trough at the lower 1/3 of the esophagus [13]. Such changes are frequently identified in patients with nonobstructive dysphagia (fig. 1) [14]. A defect or prominent trough in the pressure profile of the peristaltic wave may impair bolus transit. A wider than normal transitional zone may also cause dysphagia [15, 16]. Esophageal diverticula are often accompanied by dysphagia [17]; HRM has now revealed a defect in peristaltic contractile activity at the level of diverticulum [18] (fig. 2). A trough in the distal esophagus can be identified in some sub-

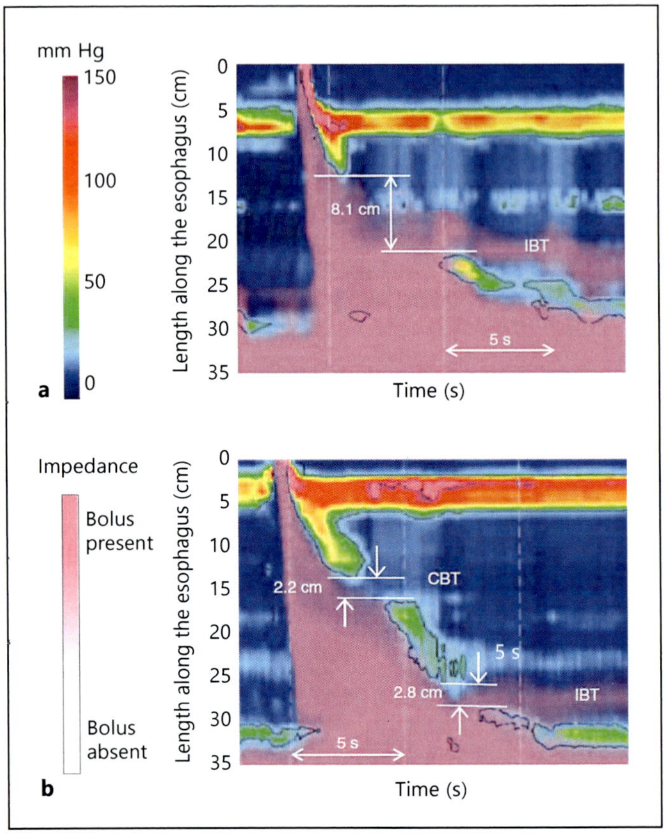

Fig. 1. Examples of incomplete bolus transit (IBT) in high-resolution impedance manometry studies attributable to large or small breaks in the 20 mm Hg isobaric contour. Impedance data are displayed by overlaid pink coloration with the pink shading indicative of areas on the topography plots with retained bolus. The associated dimensions of the critical break in the isobaric contours are indicated on each panel. **a** IBT is associated with a large proximal break in the 20 mm Hg isobaric contour. **b** The small proximal break is associated with complete bolus transit (CBT), whereas the distal break is associated with IBT. Reproduced with permission from Roman et al. [12].

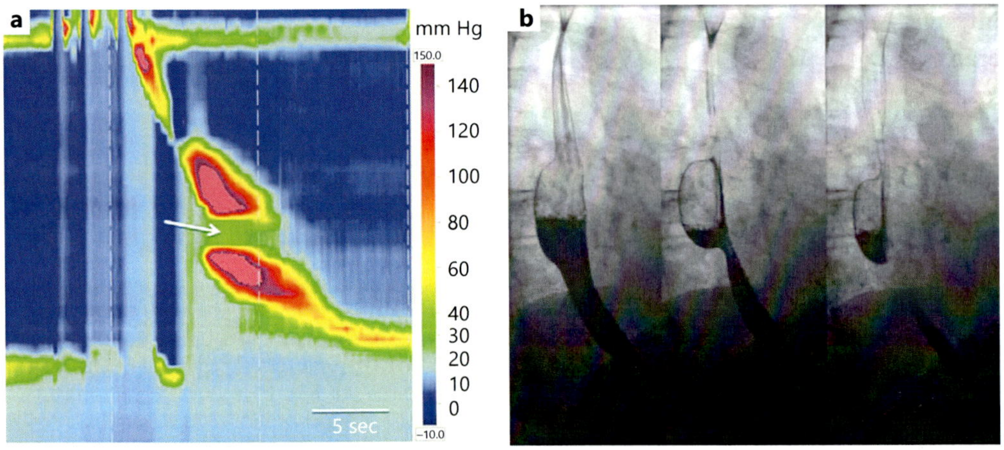

Fig. 2. HRM of a patient with a mid-esophageal diverticulum showing a pressure trough 10 cm above LES (**a**), which corresponds to findings on fluoroscopy (**b**).

Table 4. Secondary nonobstructive dysphagia and its main mechanisms

Primary disorder	Pathogenesis	Pathophysiology
Systemic sclerosis	smooth muscle degeneration of the esophagus	impaired peristaltic contractility
Eosinophilic esophagitis	eosinophilic infiltration (?)	mural rigidity (decreased distensibility)
Parkinson's disease	degenerative neural changes in the esophagus	impaired peristaltic consequence
Esophageal diverticula	muscular defect at diverticulum	interruption of peristaltic consequence

jects. Those who have a significant defect in the distal esophagus may have dysphagia and impaired bolus transport [12]. Incomplete bolus transport is observed in patients with breaks of >5 cm in the 20 mm Hg isobaric contour, and variable impairment in breaks of 2–5 cm in the 20 mm Hg contour.

Secondary Nonobstructive Dysphagia

Some diseases may cause secondary nonobstructive dysphagia through changes in esophageal smooth muscle, the mucosal layer, neural degeneration or the presence of regional muscular defects. These are summarized in table 4.

Systemic sclerosis (SSc), or scleroderma, patients have specific changes in gastrointestinal smooth muscle, especially in esophageal smooth muscle [19]. Due to degenerative changes in the esophageal smooth muscle, peristaltic contractile activities are lost in patients with SSc, who show impaired bolus transit with symptoms of dysphagia, sensation of food sticking in the esophagus, along with severe reflux esophagitis due to the loss of anti-reflux ability at the LES.

EoE is accompanied by dysphagia in most patients, both children and adults. A high prevalence of dysphagia in EoE was first reported in pediatric patients [20]. Common symptoms in patients with EoE are dysphagia (sensation of food sticking in the esophagus) and food impaction, along with reflux symptoms, both in children and in adults [1, 21–23]. Functional testing shows decreased distensibility of the esophagus through measurements of the cross-sectional area of a balloon distended in the esophagus [24]. However, decreased distensibility of the esophagus in patients with EoE does not correlate with mucosal eosinophil counts [24]. Manometric studies show ineffective esophageal motility (36%), DES (1/77) and nutcracker esophagus (1/77) in adult EoE patients [21], which is similar to nonspecific nonobstructive dysphagia, except for a lower prevalence of DES in EoE.

Parkinson's disease often induces oropharyngeal dysphagia, but also esophageal dysphagia is a common complication [25, 26]. Manometrically, 61–73% of patients have dysmotility of the esophagus, mostly repetitive simultaneous contractions or aperistalsis [25, 26]. Bolus transit is also impaired in patients with Parkinson's disease [27].

Patients with an esophageal diverticulum often complain of dysphagia [17]. The swallowed bolus may stick at the level of the diverticulum, because a defect in the muscular layer at the level of diverticulum fails to propel the bolus, which is clearly demonstrated in HRM [12, 18].

Correlation between Symptom and Objective Findings

In nonobstructive dysphagia patients with normal manometry, abnormal transit can be found in some patients [15], but its prevalence has varied widely from 18 to 100%, a variability which may reflect the small numbers of patients studied (4–17 patients in these series) [7–9, 28].

In other series of patients, similar findings are reported. In a combination of various patients referred for esophageal manometry and function studies, impaired bolus transit was observed in 4–23% of normal manometry subjects with or without the symptom of dysphagia [29, 30]. In studies among GERD patients, abnormal peristalsis and abnormal transit on impedance were more frequently found in patients with ineffective esophageal motility (IEM) than in those without IEM, but the prevalence of dysphagia as a symptom was almost equal in both groups [31]. Similarly, among patients with Parkinson's disease, dysmotility and the symptom of dysphagia do not correlate [25].

Speculative Explanation of Dysphagia with Normal Transit

Nguyen et al. [9] proposed two explanations for the occurrence of dysphagia among those with normal transit with normal manometry; none detected in manometric studies. Firstly, they proposed impaired wall compliance in the intrabolus domain that precedes the contraction wave, possibly due to an impairment of descending inhibition, as the bolus seems to travel closer to the peristaltic wave than it does in healthy volunteers. Secondly, they proposed that a deficiency in pharyngeal propulsion of the bolus impaired the rapid transport of the bolus through the esophagus.

A bolus flow resistance study showed higher resistance in NOD patients in relation to perception of bolus transit [10]; this suggests the presence of an esophageal motility disorder despite normal findings on manometric study. Decreased distensibility of the esophagus in EoE [24] may have similar mechanical characteristics to the aforementioned increased bolus flow resistance [10] and impaired wall compliance [9].

Such mural change may progress to ineffective esophageal peristalsis and/or simultaneous contractions such as DES, which also develop impaired bolus transit. Accordingly, decreased distensibility of the esophagus, currently of unknown etiology, might not only lead to the development of the symptom of dysphagia, but might ultimately culminate in both an abnormality in transit and manometric changes. Further studies to clarify our understanding of nonobstructive dysphagia are required.

Therapeutic Approaches

As the pathophysiologic mechanism of nonobstructive dysphagia has not been established, empirical therapy is applied. As the symptom suggests impaired transit of the bolus, empiric esophageal dilatation is applied to nonobstructive dysphagia patients, and a long-term efficacy of 96% was reported in response to various dilators with diameters of 17.0–17.5 mm at one year (n = 4,263) [32] and 85% in response to a 50-Fr (16.6-mm) bougie at 2 years (n = 13) [33]. This suggests that patients with nonobstructive dysphagia may have some kind of flow resistance in the esophagus.

References

1 Dellon ES, Irani AM, Hill MR, Hirano I: Development and field testing of a novel patient-reported outcome measure of dysphagia in patients with eosinophilic esophagitis. Aliment Pharmacol Ther 2013;38:634–642.

2 Mittal RK, Siskind BN, Hongo M, Flye MW, McCallum RW: Dysphagia aortica. Clinical, radiological, and manometric findings. Dig Dis Sci 1986;31:379–384.

3 Levitt B, Richter JE: Dysphagia lusoria; a comprehensive review. Dis Esophagus 2007;20;455–460.

4 Kuo P, Holloway RH, Nguyen NQ: Current and future techniques in the evaluation of dysphagia. J Gastroenterol Hepatol 2012;27:873–881.

5 Roman S, Kahrilas PJ: Challenges in the swallowing mechanism; nonobstructive dysphagia in the era of high-resolution manometry and impedance. Gastroenterol Clin North Am 2011;40:823–835.

6 Schoeman MN, Holloway RH: Secondary oesophageal peristalsis in patients with non-obstructive dysphagia. Gut 1994;35:1523–1528.

7 Conchillo JM, Nguyen NQ, Samsom M, Holloway RH, Smout AJ: Multichannel intraluminal impedance monitoring in the evaluation of patients with non-obstructive Dysphagia. Am J Gastroenterol 2005;100: 2624–2632.

8 Burgess NG, Wyeth JW: An audit of combined multichannel intraluminal impedance manometry in the assessment of dysphagia. J Gastroenterol Hepatol 2011;26(suppl 3):79–82.

9 Nguyen NQ, Holloway RH, Smout AJ, Omari TI: Automated impedance-manometry analysis detects esophageal motor dysfunction in patients who have non-obstructive dysphagia with normal manometry. Neurogastroenterol Motil 2013;25:238–245, e164.

10 Chen CL, Yi CH, Liu TT, Hsu CS, Omari TI: Characterization of esophageal pressure-flow abnormalities in patients with non-obstructive dysphagia and normal manometry findings. J Gastroenterol Hepatol 2013;28:946–953.

11 Kahrilas PJ, Dodds WJ, Hogan WJ: Effect of peristaltic dysfunction on esophageal volume clearance. Gastroenterology 1988;94:73–80.

12 Roman S, Lin Z, Kwiatek MA, Pandolfino JE, Kahrilas PJ: Weak peristalsis in esophageal pressure topography; classification and association with dysphagia. Am J Gastroenterol 2011;106:349–356.

13 Clouse RE, Staiano A: Topography of normal and high-amplitude esophageal peristalsis. Am J Physiol 1993;265:G1098–G1107.

14 Leite LP, Johnston BT, Barrett J, Castell JA, Castell DO: Ineffective esophageal motility (IEM); the primary finding in patients with nonspecific esophageal motility disorder. Dig Dis Sci 1997;42:1859–1865.

15 Bogte A, Bredenoord AJ, Oors J, Siersema PD, Smout AJ: Relationship between esophageal contraction patterns and clearance of swallowed liquid and solid boluses in healthy controls and patients with dysphagia. Neurogastroenterol Motil 2012;24: e364–e372.
16 Kumar SD, Cong X, Dziura J, Sheth AA: Transitional zone length is associated with non-obstructive dysphagia in patients with normal high resolution manometry (abstract). Gastroenterology 2011;140: S-299.
17 do Nascimento FA, Lemme EM, Costa MM: Esophageal diverticula; pathogenesis, clinical aspects, and natural history. Dysphagia 2006;21:198–205.
18 De Schepper HU, Smout AJ, Bredenoord AJ: An unusual cause of dysphagia. Clin Gastroenterol Hepatol 2013;11:A20.
19 Sjogren RW: Gastrointestinal motility disorders in scleroderma. Arthritis Rheum 1994;37:1265–1282.
20 Khan S, Orenstein SR, Di Lorenzo C, Kocoshis SA, Putnam PE, Sigurdsson L, Shalaby TM: Eosinophilic esophagitis; strictures, impactions, dysphagia. Dig Dis Sci 2003;48:22–29.
21 Furuta GT, Liacouras CA, Collins MH, Gupta SK, Justinich C, Putnam PE, Bonis P, Hassall E, Straumann A, Rothenberg ME, First International Gastrointestinal Eosinophil Research Symposium (FIGERS) Subcommittees: Eosinophilic esophagitis in children and adults; a systematic review and consensus recommendations for diagnosis and treatment. Gastroenterology 2007;133:1342–1363.
22 Nicodème F, Hirano I, Chen J, Robinson K, Lin Z, Xiao Y, Gonsalves N, Kwasny MJ, Kahrilas PJ, Pandolfino JE: Esophageal distensibility as a measure of disease severity in patients with eosinophilic esophagitis. Clin Gastroenterol Hepatol 2013;11:1101–1107.
23 Prasad GA, Talley NJ, Romero Y, Arora AS, Kryzer LA, Smyrk TC, Alexander JA: Prevalence and predictive factors of eosinophilic esophagitis in patients presenting with dysphagia; a prospective study. Am J Gastroenterol 2007;102:2627–2632.
24 Kwiatek MA, Hirano I, Kahrilas PJ, Rothe J, Luger D, Pandolfino JE: Mechanical properties of the esophagus in eosinophilic esophagitis. Gastroenterology 2011;140:82–90.
25 Castell JA, Johnston BT, Colcher A, Li Q, Gideon RM, Castell DO: Manometric abnormalities of the oesophagus in patients with Parkinson's disease. Neurogastroenterol Motil 2001;13:361–364.
26 Bassotti G, Germani U, Pagliaricci S, Plesa A, Giulietti O, Mannarino E, Morelli A: Esophageal manometric abnormalities in Parkinson's disease. Dysphagia 1998;13:28–31.
27 Potulska A, Friedman A, Królicki L, Spychala A: Swallowing disorders in Parkinson's disease. Parkinsonism Relat Disord 2003;9:349–353.
28 Chen CL, Yi CH: Clinical correlates of dysphagia to oesophageal dysmotility; studies using combined manometry and impedance. Neurogastroenterol Motil 2008;20:611–617.
29 Tutuian R, Castell DO: Combined multichannel intraluminal impedance and manometry clarifies esophageal function abnormalities; study in 350 patients. Am J Gastroenterol 2004;99:1011–1109.
30 Koya DL, Agrawal A, Freeman JE, Castell DO: Impedance detected abnormal bolus transit in patients with normal esophageal manometry. Sensitive indicator of esophageal functional abnormality? Dis Esophagus 2008;21:563–569.
31 Lazarescu A, Karamanolis G, Aprile L, De Oliveira RB, Dantas R, Sifrim D: Perception of dysphagia; lack of correlation with objective measurements of esophageal function. Neurogastroenterol Motil 2010;22:1292–1297, e336–e337.
32 Colon VJ, Young MA, Ramirez FC: The short- and long-term efficacy of empirical esophageal dilation in patients with nonobstructive dysphagia: a prospective, randomized study. Am J Gastroenterol 2000;95:910–913.
33 Olson JS, Lieberman DA, Sonnenberg A: Empiric dilation in non-obstructive dysphagia. Dig Dis Sci 2008;53:1192–1197.

Michio Hongo, MD, PhD
Kurokawa General Hospital
60 Nishi-Hinoki, Yoshioka, Taiwa
Kurokawa, Miyagi 981-3682 (Japan)
E-Mail m-hongo@med.tohoku.ac.jp

Quigley EMM, Hongo M, Fukudo S (eds): Functional and GI Motility Disorders.
Front Gastrointest Res. Basel, Karger, 2014, vol 33, pp 25–37 (DOI: 10.1159/000356734)

Gastroparesis

Henry P. Parkman

Gastroenterology Section, Temple University School of Medicine, Philadelphia, Pa., USA

Abstract

Gastroparesis is a chronic symptomatic disorder of the stomach characterized by delayed emptying without evidence of mechanical obstruction. Symptoms from gastroparesis include nausea, vomiting, early satiety, postprandial fullness, and, in some patients, upper abdominal pain. The three main causes are diabetic, postsurgical, and idiopathic. Management of gastroparesis includes assessment and correction of dehydration and malnutrition if present, maintaining nutritional intake, relief of symptoms, improvement of gastric emptying and, in diabetics, glycemic control. Nutritional state should be managed by oral dietary modifications. Medical treatment entails use of prokinetic and antiemetic therapies. For refractory cases, jejunostomy feeding tube, gastric electric stimulator, and pyloromyotomy may need to be considered. Unfortunately, current approved treatment options do not adequately address clinical need. Attention should be given to the development of new effective therapies for symptomatic control.

Gastroparesis is a chronic symptomatic disorder of the stomach manifested by delayed emptying without evidence of mechanical obstruction [1]. This classic motility disorder of the stomach can lead to marked dysfunction in patients with poor quality of life. Although in many patients symptoms can be controlled with medical therapy, some patients remain markedly symptomatic with progressive weight loss. This chapter provides an overview of gastroparesis and updates the present status of our understanding of this disorder and the treatments available.

Epidemiology

Gastroparesis occurs more often in women than men. Interestingly, this is true for the three main forms of gastroparesis: idiopathic, diabetic, and even postsurgical. The epidemiology of gastroparesis, however, has not been systematically studied. This stems from the fact that for proper diagnosis a gastric emptying test is needed, something that presently cannot be done in population studies. Data from the Rochester Epidemiology Project, a database of linked medical records of residents of Olmsted County, Minnesota, show that the age-adjusted incidence of definite gastroparesis per 100,000 person-years for the years 1996–2006 was 9.8 for women and 2.4 for men [2]. Definite gastroparesis was defined as a diagnosis of delayed gastric emptying by standard scintigraphy and symptoms of nausea and/or vomiting, postprandial fullness, early satiety, bloating, or epigastric pain for more than 3 months. The age-adjusted prevalence of definite gastroparesis per 100,000 persons was 37.8 for women and 9.6 for men. More recent estimates have suggested that these prevalence rates for gastroparesis were an underestimation and that the prevalence is higher, approaching 2% of the general population [3].

The prevalence of gastroparesis might be increasing. Data from the US Healthcare Cost and Utilization Project (HCUP) Nationwide Inpatient Sample (NIS), a nationally representative sample of 5–8 million hospitalizations per year, show that, from 1995 to 2004, hospitalizations with gastroparesis as the primary diagnosis increased by 158% and those with gastroparesis as the secondary diagnosis increased by 136% compared with a 13% increase in all hospitalizations [3]. Of the 5 upper gastrointestinal conditions studied as primary diagnoses (i.e. gastroparesis, gastroesophageal reflux disease, gastric ulcer, gastritis, nonspecific nausea/vomiting), gastroparesis had the longest length of stay and the second highest total charges in 1995 and 2004. The increase in hospitalization rate for gastroparesis has occurred since the year 2000, and could reflect increasing prevalence and/or the effects of heightened awareness about, and better identification of, gastroparesis [4]. This increase in gastroparesis hospitalizations may also be due, in part, to the increasing rate of diabetes leading to more cases of diabetic gastroparesis, withdrawal of some gastroparesis treatments from the market (cisapride, tegaserod) with hospitalizations resulting from symptoms not being adequately treated, and hospitalizations needed for insertion of the gastric electric stimulator.

Symptoms

Common symptoms of gastroparesis include nausea (>90% of patients), vomiting (84% of patients), and early satiety (60% of patients) [5]. Other symptoms include postprandial fullness and abdominal pain [6, 7]. Symptoms can be persistent or can manifest as episodic flares. Weight loss, malnutrition, and dehydration may be prominent in severe cases. In diabetics, gastroparesis may adversely affect glycemic control.

Symptom profile can be established, and symptom severity assessed with the Gastroparesis Cardinal Symptom Index (GCSI), a subset of the Patient Assessment of Upper Gastrointestinal Symptoms (PAGI-SYM) [8]. The GCSI comprises 3 subscales (nausea and vomiting, postprandial fullness and early satiety, and bloating) that the patient scores with reference to the preceding 2 weeks [8]. A variant on the GCSI, the GCSI daily diary can be used to record symptoms on a daily basis and may be more accurate in recording symptoms [9].

Although it has been a common assumption that the aforementioned gastrointestinal symptoms can be attributed to a delay in gastric emptying, most investigations have observed only weak correlations between symptom severity and the degree of gastric stasis. In general, the symptoms that appear to be best correlated with a delay in gastric emptying include nausea, vomiting, early satiety, and postprandial fullness [10, 11]. Some symptoms that have been described in patients with gastroparesis, such as bloating and upper abdominal pain, are not correlated with delayed gastric emptying and might be related to sensory alterations and also be present in patients with gastroparesis.

Etiology

Major etiologies of gastroparesis are diabetic, postsurgical, and idiopathic [1, 12, 13]. Less common causes of gastroparesis include connective tissue disease, neurologic diseases such as Parkinson's disease, eating disorders, metabolic or endocrine conditions (hypothyroidism), critical illness, and medications such as opiates, anticholinergics and calcium channel blockers [12]. In addition, GP-1 analogs, such as exenatide, used in the treatment of type 2 diabetes mellitus, can delay gastric emptying [1].

Gastroparesis is a relatively common complication of diabetes: delayed gastric emptying has been found to occur in approximately 40% of patients with longstanding type 1 diabetes and approximately 20% of patients with type 2 diabetes [12]. These estimates come from academic medical centers, and true estimates may be lower in the general population and among patients seeing primary care physicians. Diabetic gastroparesis is often attributed to chronic hyperglycemia-induced damage to the vagus nerve and is frequently observed in association with other diabetic complications such as neuropathy, retinopathy, and nephropathy. Glucose can modify gastric emptying tests and symptoms: hyperglycemia can delay gastric emptying and worsen symptoms of gastroparesis, whereas hypoglycemia may accelerate gastric emptying.

Postsurgical gastroparesis can occur with many types of operations, but is most often observed after upper abdominal procedures because of injury to, or division of the vagus nerve [1]. In the past, surgical procedures for peptic ulcer disease, such as antrectomy with vagotomy, were associated with the development of gastroparesis. However, this type of surgery is performed less often nowadays due to the use of proton pump inhibitors and treatments for *Helicobacter pylori*. Currently, Nissen fundoplication is probably the surgical procedure most commonly associated with gastroparesis. Bariatric surgeries and pancreatic surgery have also been associated with gastroparesis.

Idiopathic gastroparesis, with no obvious cause for the gastroparesis, is a commonly used descriptor for some patients with gastroparesis. The characteristics of 243 patients with idiopathic gastroparesis enrolled in the National Institute of Diabetes and Digestive and Kidney Diseases Gastroparesis Clinical Research Consortium Registry were recently described based on medical histories, symptom questionnaires, and gastric emptying scintigraphy [14]. The mean age of these patients was 41 years, and the majority (88%) was female. Half (50%) had an acute onset of symptoms. The most common presenting symptoms were nausea (34%), vomiting (19%), and abdominal pain (23%). Severe delay in gastric emptying (>35% retention at 4 h) was present in 28% of patients. Severe delay in gastric emptying was associated with more severe symptoms of nausea and vomiting and loss of appetite compared with patients with mild or moderate delay. The percentages of patients with severe anxiety and severe depression were 36 and 18%, respectively; 86% met the criteria for functional dyspepsia; predominantly, the postprandial distress syndrome. Thus, idiopathic gastroparesis is a heterogeneous syndrome that primarily affects young women and often affects overweight or obese individuals.

A minority of patients with idiopathic gastroparesis (19% in the National Institute of Diabetes and Digestive and Kidney Diseases Gastroparesis Clinical Research Consortium Registry study above [14]) report an initial infectious prodrome such as gastroenteritis or respiratory infection. It has been suggested that idiopathic gastroparesis of acute onset with infectious prodrome could constitute postviral or viral injury to the neural innervation of the stomach or the interstitial cells of Cajal in the stomach. In some series, patients with postviral gastroparesis improve over time, generally over several years.

Pathophysiology

Gastric emptying is mediated by the vagus nerve, which helps regulate fundic accommodation, antral contraction, and pyloric relaxation [1]. These regional gastric motility changes with food ingestion are then mediated through smooth muscle cells, which control stomach contractions; interstitial cells of Cajal, which regulate gastric pacemaker activity, and enteric neurons, which initiate smooth muscle cell activity [1]. The pathophysiology of gastroparesis has not been fully elucidated but appears to involve abnormalities in the function of several elements including the autonomic nervous system, smooth muscle cells, enteric neurons, and interstitial cells of Cajal. Histologic studies demonstrate defects in the morphology of enteric neurons, smooth muscle cells, and interstitial cells of Cajal and increased concentrations of inflammatory cells in gastric tissue [1, 12, 13].

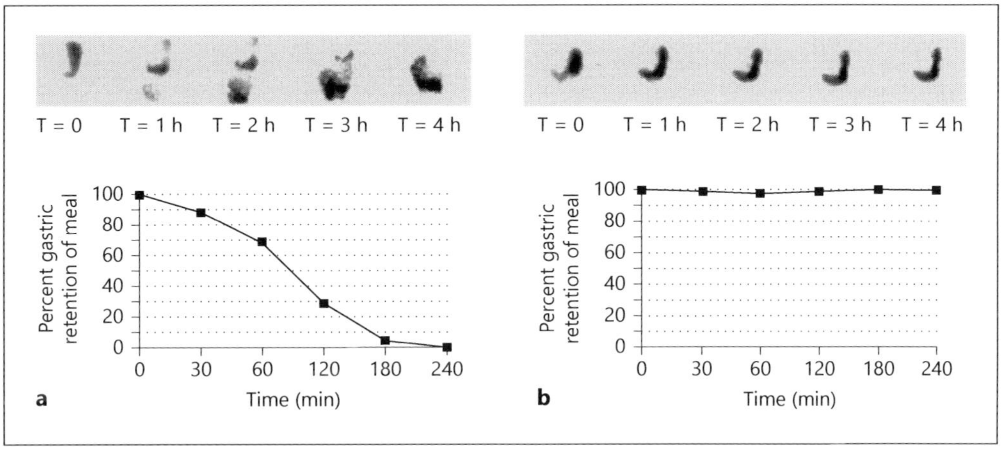

Fig. 1. Illustrations of normal (**a**) and delayed (**b**) gastric emptying rate (percent gastric retention of meal) after a low-fat egg white sandwich meal with water. Image courtesy of Drs. Henry Parkman and Alan Maurer.

Diagnosis

The differential diagnosis of gastroparesis entails excluding other possible causes including peptic ulcer disease, gastric outlet obstruction, neoplasm, and small bowel obstruction [12]. For the evaluation of these, an upper endoscopy should be performed.

For evaluating gastric emptying, the standard test is gastric emptying scintigraphy, which uses a labeled isotope bound to solid food to image gastric emptying [12, 15]. The methodology used varies considerably between different centers. Standardization of gastric emptying among different centers has been suggested using a 4-hour imaging protocol with scans taken 0, 1, 2, 4 h after ingestion of a radioactive Tc-99m-labeled low-fat egg white with jam and 2 pieces of toast. Examples of normal and delayed gastric emptying rates measured with gastric emptying scintigraphy after consumption of a low-fat egg white sandwich meal with water are shown in figure 1.

Use of the wireless motility capsule to quantify luminal pH and pressure is an alternative to gastric emptying scintigraphy [12]. This test also measures whole-gut transit – that is, gastric emptying, small bowel transit, and colonic transit. Gastric emptying is manifested by a sharp increase in pH representing the capsule passing from the acidic stomach to the alkaline small intestine.

Breath tests for gastric emptying, another alternative to gastric emptying scintigraphy, measure labeled nonradioactive $^{13}CO_2$ in exhaled breath samples after ingestion of a $^{13}CO_2$-labeled meal. Breath samples are obtained periodically over several hours. The appearance of $^{13}CO_2$ in the breath represents the net effects of gastric emptying, duodenal absorption, hepatic metabolism and pulmonary excretion where gastric emptying is the rate-limiting step [12]. Findings generally correlate well with results of gastric emptying scintigraphy. This test is used clinically in Europe, whereas in the United States, breath tests are most often employed in research studies and rarely used in the clinic.

Gastric emptying testing is useful in diagnosing gastroparesis. There are several drawbacks. First, gastric emptying rates generally correlate poorly with symptoms and the quality of life impact of gastroparesis [16, 17]. This finding suggests that factors, in addition to slow gastric emptying, contribute to symptoms. Second, relatively high interindividual and intraindividual variability in gastric emptying rates constitutes another limitation of gastric motility testing [12]. The relative contributions to this variability of test methodology and biologic inconsistency in gastric emptying are currently not known.

Management

Management of gastroparesis is guided by the goals of correcting fluid, electrolyte, and nutritional deficiencies, identifying and treating the cause of delayed gastric emptying (e.g. diabetes), and suppressing or eliminating symptoms [1]. Care of patients generally relies on dietary modification, medications that stimulate gastric motor activity, and antiemetic drug therapy.

Dietary Treatment

Dietary measures entail adjustment to meal composition and frequency [1, 12]. Eating small meals is recommended as patients often have early satiety, that is feeling full when eating a normal-size meal; in addition, larger meals may alter gastric emptying times. Consuming mainly liquids such as soups can be useful as gastric emptying of liquids is often preserved in patients with gastroparesis [1]. Avoidance of fats and indigestible fibers is recommended because they delay gastric emptying [1, 12]. When small meals are used in the gastroparesis diet, more frequent meals, 3 meals per day plus 2 snack type meals are often needed to maintain caloric intake.

Glucose Control in Diabetic Patients

Diabetic patients with gastroparesis frequently exhibit labile blood glucose concentrations with prolonged periods of significant hyperglycemia. Hyperglycemia itself can delay gastric emptying. Hyperglycemia can counteract the accelerating effects of prokinetic agents on gastric emptying. Improvement of glucose control increases antral contractility, corrects gastric dysrhythmias, and accelerates emptying. To date, there have been no long-term studies confirming the beneficial effects of maintenance of near euglycemia on gastroparetic symptoms. Nevertheless, the consistent findings of physiologic studies in healthy volunteers and diabetic patients provide a compelling argument to strive for near-normal blood glucose levels in affected diabetic patients. Generally, patients give their meal time insulin after ingesting the meal, to ensure that the entire anticipated meal is actually consumed and without vomiting.

Prokinetic Agents

Medications with gastric prokinetic properties, which are the mainstay of treatment for gastroparesis, include metoclopramide, erythromycin, and domperidone [1, 14, 15, 18]. Intravenous agents currently available to treat hospitalized patients include metoclopramide and erythromycin. Several prokinetic agents are being studied for patients with gastroparesis; these include newer 5-HT_4 receptor agonists with less cardiac side effects, newer motilin receptor agonists with less evidence of tachyphylaxis and without antibiotic properties, and newer ghrelin receptor agonists.

Metoclopramide

Metoclopramide, a substituted benzamide structurally related to procainamide, exhibits both prokinetic and antiemetic actions. The drug is a dopamine type 2 receptor antagonist both in the CNS and in the stomach. Metoclopramide also has $5HT_3$ receptor antagonist activity that might also provide an antiemetic effect. In addition, it has some $5HT_4$ agonist activity releasing acetylcholine from intrinsic myenteric cholinergic neurons that might help enhance gastric emptying. The prokinetic properties of metoclopramide are limited primarily to the stomach. Reglan can cause both acute and chronic CNS side effects in some patients. These side effects should be discussed with the patient prior to treatment and documented in the patient's medical record. In the United States, metoclopramide is approved for diabetic gastroparesis for up to 12 weeks' duration. Patients with gastroparesis have chronic nausea and often need longer periods of treatment. Recently, in Europe, it has been suggested that metoclopramide be used for only several days' duration for acute treatment of chemotherapy-induced vomiting.

Erythromycin

The macrolide antibiotic erythromycin exerts prokinetic effects via action on gastroduodenal receptors for motilin, an endogenous peptide responsible for initiation of the MMC in the upper gut. When administered exogenously, motilin stimulates antral contractility and elicits premature antroduodenal phase III activity. Erythromycin produces effects on gastroduodenal motility similar to motilin.

Clinically, erythromycin has been shown to stimulate gastric emptying in diabetic gastroparesis, idiopathic gastroparesis, and postvagotomy gastroparesis. Erythromycin may be most potent when used intravenously; it is often used to clear the stomach of blood prior to an upper endoscopy in a patient with upper gastrointestinal bleeding. Limited data exist concerning the clinical efficacy of erythromycin in reducing symptoms of gastroparesis. In a systematic review of studies on oral erythromycin with symptom assessment as a clinical end point, improvement was noted in 43% of patients [19]. One study comparing erythromycin and metoclopramide in an open-label, crossover fashion in diabetic gastroparesis found similar efficacy [20].

Oral administration of erythromycin should be initiated at low doses (e.g. 125–250 mg 3 or 4 times daily). Liquid suspension erythromycin may be preferred because it is rapidly and more reliably absorbed. Intravenous erythromycin (100 mg every 8 h) is used for inpatients hospitalized for severe refractory gastroparesis. Side effects of erythromycin at higher doses include nausea, vomiting, and abdominal pain. Because these symptoms may mimic those of gastroparesis, erythromycin may have a narrow therapeutic window in some patients. There is a report that erythromycin chronically may be associated with higher mortality from cardiac disease, especially when combined with agents that inhibit cytochrome p-450, such as calcium channel blockers [21]. Similar concerns have been raised in relation to azithromycin which has been suggested as an alternative oral macrolide [22].

Domperidone

The effects of domperidone on the upper gut are similar to those of metoclopramide, including stimulation of antral contractions and promotion of antroduodenal coordination. In addition to prokinetic actions in the stomach, domperidone exhibits antiemetic properties via actions on the area postrema, a brainstem region with a porous blood-brain barrier. Domperidone does not readily cross the blood-brain barrier; therefore, it is much less likely to cause extrapyramidal side effects than metoclopramide. Side effects to domperidone include breast lactation, headaches, and palpitations. Domperidone has been associated with prolongation of the cardiac QTc interval and sudden cardiac death [23, 24].

The FDA has developed a program for physicians who would like to prescribe domperidone for their patients with severe upper GI motility disorders that are refractory to standard therapy to open an Investigational New Drug Application (IND). An IND is a request for FDA authorization to administer an investigational drug to humans. Such authorization would allow the importation, interstate shipment, and administration of the drug even though it is not approved for sale in the US. Use of this IND mechanism for use of domperidone also will require institutional review board approval. An EKG and blood work to check potassium and magnesium are obtained prior to starting domperidone; these are repeated after 4–8 weeks of treatment.

Antiemetic Medications

Antiemetic agents are given acutely for symptomatic nausea and vomiting. The principal classes of drugs that have been used for symptomatic treatment of nausea and vomiting are phenothiazines, antihistamines, anticholinergics, dopamine receptor antagonists, and, more recently, serotonin receptor antagonists. The antiemetic action of phenothiazine compounds appears to be mediated primarily through a central antidopaminergic mechanism in the area postrema of the brain. Commonly used agents include prochlorperazine (Compazine), trimethobenzamide (Tigan), and promethazine (Phenergan).

Serotonin (5-HT_3) receptor antagonists, such as ondansetron (Zofran) and granisetron (Kytril), have been shown to be helpful in treating or preventing chemotherapy-induced nausea and vomiting. The primary site of action of these compounds is probably the chemoreceptor trigger zone since there is a high density of 5-HT_3 receptors in the area postrema. Ondansetron is now frequently used for nausea and vomiting related to a variety of other etiologies. These drugs are best given on a p.r.n. basis due to their cost. Emend (aprepitant) is a recently approved substance P/neurokinin 1 receptor antagonist for chemotherapy-induced nausea and vomiting. It has not been studied in other forms of nausea and vomiting, such as gastroparesis.

Antiemetics include the phenothiazine derivatives (e.g. prochlorperazine), the serotonin-3 receptor antagonists (e.g. ondansetron), the dopamine receptor antagonists (e.g. metoclopramide), the histamine receptor antagonists (e.g. diphenhydramine), and benzodiazepines (e.g. lorazepam) [1, 18].

Refractory Patients with Gastroparesis

Patients with refractory gastroparesis need treatment at a variety of levels directed at nutritional care, prokinetic medications, antiemetic therapies, pain control, glycemic control, and, often, psychological measures. Surgical and endoscopic approaches are considered in patients in whom drug therapy is ineffective and who cannot meet their nutritional requirements [1]. Surgical treatments include placement of jejunostomy tubes and gastric electrical stimulation [1]. These options are typically considered only in patients with severe, refractory gastroparesis.

Combination Therapy

In moderately to severely symptomatic patients, therapy with both a prokinetic agent and antiemetic agent is often needed. Prokinetic agents act via different mechanisms to enhance gastric emptying. Theoretically, the addition of a second prokinetic agent may augment the response to the first drug if the two agents act on different receptor subtypes. Dual prokinetic therapy with domperidone and cisapride has been reported to accelerate emptying and reduce symptoms in some patients with refractory gastroparesis. Combinations of available prokinetic agents in the United States, such as metoclopramide and erythromycin, or domperidone and erythromycin, have not been specifically studied. Since metoclopramide and domperidone are both D_2 receptor antagonists, these should not be used together.

Pyloric Botulinum Toxin Injection

Gastric emptying is a highly regulated process reflecting the integration of the propulsive forces of proximal fundic tone and distal antral contractions with the functional resistance provided by the pylorus. Manometric studies of patients with diabetic gastroparesis have shown, in some patients, prolonged periods of increased pyloric tone and phasic contractions, a phenomenon termed pylorospasm [25]. Botulinum toxin is a potent inhibitor of acetylcholine neuromuscular transmission and has been used to treat spastic somatic muscle disorders as well as achalasia. Several studies have tested the effects of pyloric injection of botulinum toxin in patients with diabetic and idiopathic gastroparesis [1]. Initial studies were unblinded in small numbers of patients from single centers and have observed mild improvements in gastric emptying and modest reductions in symptoms for several months. Two double-blind studies have been reported; these show an improvement in gastric emptying, but no effect on symptoms compared to placebo [26]. Endoscopic treatment entails injection of botulinum toxin (Botox; Allergan Inc.) into the pyloric sphincter. Thus, botulinum toxin injections do not result in sustained improvement in symptoms of gastroparesis.

Psychotropic Medications as Symptom Modulators

Tricyclic antidepressants may have significant benefits in suppressing symptoms in some patients with nausea and vomiting as well as patients with abdominal pain. Doses of tricyclic antidepressants used are lower than used to treat depression. A reasonable starting dose for a tricyclic drug is 10–25 mg at bedtime. If benefit is not observed in several weeks, doses are increased by 10- to 25-mg increments up to 50–100 mg. Side effects are common with use of tricyclic antidepressants and can interfere with management and lead to a change in medication in 25% of patients. The secondary amines, nortriptyline and desipramine, may have fewer side effects. The recent NIH gastroparesis consortium study with nortriptyline in idiopathic gastroparesis did not show an effect on overall symptoms of gastroparesis

[27]. However, there was a suggestion that low doses of nortriptyline might decrease nausea, whereas higher doses might decrease fullness. There are limited data on the use of selective serotonin reuptake inhibitors in gastroparesis or functional dyspepsia.

Gastric Electric Stimulation

Gastric electric stimulation is a treatment for refractory gastroparesis [28]. It involves an implantable neurostimulator that delivers a high-frequency (12 cpm), low-energy signal with short pulses. With this device, stimulating wires are sutured into the gastric muscle along the greater curvature during laparoscopy or laparotomy. These leads are attached to the electric stimulator, which is positioned in a subcutaneous abdominal pouch. Based on the initial studies that showed symptom benefit, especially in patients with diabetic gastroparesis, the gastric electric neurostimulator was granted humanitarian approval from the FDA for the treatment of chronic, refractory nausea and vomiting secondary to idiopathic or diabetic gastroparesis. The main complication of the implantable neurostimulator has been infection, which has necessitated device removal in approximately 5% of cases. More recently, a small minority of patients have reported a 'shocking' sensation. Symptoms of nausea and vomiting can improve with stimulation; however, abdominal pain often does not [29]. The symptomatic benefit occurs more often in diabetic gastroparesis than in idiopathic gastroparesis. Further investigation is needed to confirm, firstly, the effectiveness of gastric stimulation in long-term blinded studies, and, secondly, provide such important clinical information as which patients are likely to respond, the optimal electrode position, and the optimal stimulation parameters; none of these has been rigorously evaluated to date. Future improvements may include devices that sequentially stimulate the stomach in a peristaltic sequence to promote gastric emptying.

Other Surgical Treatments for Persistently Refractory Gastroparesis Patients

Other treatments include feeding jejunostomy for nutritional support with a jejunostomy tube that bypasses the affected stomach for feedings. Venting gastrostomy tubes have been tried with success in some patients. Recently, pyloromyotomy has reemerged as a treatment for patients with gastroparesis. Gastrojejunostomy has been performed in the past with limited success. Gastric bypass with gastrojejunostomy has been used by several centers to treat gastroparesis. Partial gastrectomy should be used rarely, and only in carefully selected patients. In postsurgical gastroparesis, occasionally completion gastrectomy is performed for persistent gastroparetic symptoms.

Conclusions

Gastroparesis is identified through the recognition of the clinical symptoms and documentation of delayed gastric emptying. Management of gastroparesis includes assessment and correction of nutritional state, relief of symptoms, improvement of gastric emptying and, in diabetics, glycemic control. Patient nutritional state should be managed by oral dietary modifications. Medical treatment entails use of prokinetic and antiemetic therapies. Unfortunately, current approved treatment options do not adequately address clinical need. Attention should be given to the development of new effective therapies for symptomatic control.

References

1 Camilleri M, Parkman HP, Shafi MA, Abell TL, Gerson L: Clinical guideline: management of gastroparesis. Am J Gastroenterol 2013;108:18–37.
2 Jung HK, Choung RS, Locke GR III, et al: The incidence, prevalence, and outcomes of patients with gastroparesis in Olmsted County, Minnesota, from 1996 to 2006. Gastroenterology 2009;136:1225–1233.
3 Rey E, Choung RS, Schleck CD, et al: Prevalence of hidden gastroparesis in the community: the gastroparesis 'iceberg'. J Neurogastroenterol Motil 2012; 18:34–42.
4 Wang YR, Fisher RS, Parkman HP: Gastroparesis-related hospitalizations in the United States: trends, characteristics, and outcomes, 1995–2004. Am J Gastroenterol 2008;103:313–322.
5 Soykan I, Sivri B, Sarosiek I, Kiernan B, McCallum RW: Demography, clinical characteristics, psychological and abuse profiles, treatment, and long-term follow-up of patients with gastroparesis. Dig Dis Sci 1998;43:2398–2404.
6 Cherian D, Sachdeva P, Fisher RS, Parkman HP: Abdominal pain is a frequent symptom of gastroparesis. Clin Gastroenterol Hepatol 2010;8:676–681.
7 Hasler WL, Wilson LA, Parkman HP, et al: Bloating in gastroparesis: severity, impact, and associated factors. Am J Gastroenterol 2011;106:1492–1502.
8 Revicki DA, Rentz AM, Dubois D, et al: Development and validation of a patient-assessed gastroparesis symptom severity measure: the Gastroparesis Cardinal Symptom Index. Aliment Pharmacol Ther 2003;18:141–150.
9 Revicki DA, Camilleri M, Kuo B, et al: Development and content validity of a gastroparesis cardinal symptom index daily diary. Aliment Pharmacol Ther 2009;30:670–680.
10 Pathikonda M, Sachdeva P, Malhotra N, Fisher RS, Maurer AH, Parkman HP: Gastric emptying scintigraphy: is four hours necessary? J Clin Gastroenterol 2012;46:209–215.
11 Cassilly DW, Wang YR, Friedenberg FK, Nelson DB, Maurer AH, Parkman HP: Symptoms of gastroparesis: use of the gastroparesis cardinal symptom index in symptomatic patients referred for gastric emptying scintigraphy. Digestion 2008;78:144–151.
12 Hasler WL: Gastroparesis: pathogenesis, diagnosis, and management. Nat Rev Gastroenterol Hepatol 2011;8:438–453.
13 Hasler WL: Gastroparesis – current concepts and considerations. Medscape J Med 2008;10:16.
14 Parkman HP, Yates K, Hasler WL, et al: Clinical features of idiopathic gastroparesis vary with sex, body mass, symptom onset, delay in gastric emptying, and gastroparesis severity. Gastroenterology 2011;140: 101–115.
15 Parkman HP: Assessment of gastric emptying and small-bowel motility: scintigraphy, breath tests, manometry, and SmartPill. Gastrointest Endosc Clin N Am 2009;19:49–55.
16 Horowitz M, Maddox AF, Wishart JM, Harding PE, Chatterton BE, Shearman DJ: Relationships between oesophageal transit and solid and liquid gastric emptying in diabetes mellitus. Eur J Nucl Med 1991;18: 229–234.
17 Pasricha PJ, Colvin R, Yates K, et al: Characteristics of patients with chronic unexplained nausea and vomiting and normal gastric emptying. Clin Gastroenterol Hepatol 2011;9:567–576.e1–e4.
18 McCallum RW, George SJ: Gastric dysmotility and gastroparesis. Curr Treat Options Gastroenterol 2001;4:179–191.
19 Maganti K, Onyemere K, Jones MP: Oral erythromycin and symptomatic relief of gastroparesis: a systematic review. Am J Gastroenterol 2003;98:259–263.

20 Erbas T, Varoglu E, Erbas B, Tastekin G, Akalin S: Comparison of metoclopramide and erythromycin in the treatment of diabetic gastroparesis. Diabetes Care 1993;16:1511–1514.
21 Ray WA, Murray KT, Meredith S, Narasimhulu SS, Hall K, Stein CM: Oral erythromycin use and the risk of sudden cardiac death. N Engl J Med 2004;351: 1089–1096.
22 Mosholder AD, Mathew J, Alexander JJ, Smith H, Nambiar S: Cardiovascular risks with azithromycin and other antibacterial drugs. N Engl J Med 2013; 368:1665–1668.
23 Rossi M, Giorgi G: Domperidone and long QT syndrome. Curr Drug Saf 2010;5:257–262.
24 van Noord C, Dieleman JP, van Herpen G, Verhamme K, Sturkenboom MC: Domperidone and ventricular arrhythmia or sudden cardiac death: a population-based case-control study in the Netherlands. Drug Saf 2010;33:1003–1014.
25 Mearin F, Camilleri M, Malagelada JR: Pyloric dysfunction in diabetics with recurrent nausea and vomiting. Gastroenterology 1986;90:1919–1925.
26 Bai Y, Xu MJ, Yang X, Xu C, Gao J, Zou DW, Li ZS: A systematic review on intrapyloric botulinum toxin injection for gastroparesis. Digestion 2010;81:27–34.
27 Parkman HP, van Natta M, Abell TL, McCallum RW, Sarosiek I, Nguyen LAB, Snape WJ, Koch KL, Hasler WL, Farrugia G, Lee LA, Unalp A, Tonascia J, Hamilton FA, Pasricha PJ: GpCEC Consortium. Nortriptyline for idiopathic gastroparesis: a multicenter, randomized, double-masked, placebo-controlled trial. Gastroenterology 2013;144:A-2.
28 Abell T, McCallum R, Hocking M, Koch K, Abrahamsson H, Leblanc I, Lindberg G, Konturek J, Nowak T, Quigley EM, Tougas G, Starkebaum W: Gastric electrical stimulation for medically refractory gastroparesis. Gastroenterology 2003;125:421–428.
29 McCallum RW, Sarosiek I, Parkman HP, Snape W, Brody F, Wo J, Nowak T: Gastric electrical stimulation with Enterra therapy improves symptoms of idiopathic gastroparesis. Neurogastroenterol Motil 2013;25:815-e636.

Henry P. Parkman, MD
GI Section – Parkinson Pavilion 8th Floor, Temple University School of Medicine
3401 North Broad Street
Philadelphia, PA 19140 (USA)
E-Mail henry.parkman@temple.edu

Quigley EMM, Hongo M, Fukudo S (eds): Functional and GI Motility Disorders.
Front Gastrointest Res. Basel, Karger, 2014, vol 33, pp 38–44 (DOI: 10.1159/000356737)

The Role of Gastric Sensorineural Dysfunction in Functional Dyspepsia

Jan Tack

Translational Research Center for Gastrointestinal Disorders (TARGID), University of Leuven, Leuven, Belgium

Abstract

Visceral hypersensitivity is an attractive pathophysiological concept in functional dyspepsia (FD) and other functional disorders. Gastric barostat studies have established that a subset of FD patients are hypersensitive to gastric balloon distention. Mechanistic and pharmacological studies support the concept that gastric mechanoreceptors which respond to changes in wall tension transduce the sensitivity to gastric balloon distention, and that wide-range, low-threshold afferents are involved in conveying these signals to the central nervous system and inducing symptom perception. Both central (altered processing in pain modulatory brain centers) and peripheral (altered mucosal permeability, low-grade mucosal inflammation and changes in circulating immune cells) mechanisms may contribute to the process of visceral hypersensitivity. Relaxation of gastric smooth muscle is one approach to decrease activation of tension-sensitive mechanoreceptors, thereby decreasing symptom generation in FD.

Functional dyspepsia (FD), one of the most prevalent gastrointestinal disorders, is characterized by symptoms thought to originate from the gastroduodenal region, in the absence of organic disease that readily explains them [1]. The Rome III consensus proposed to subdivide FD into epigastric pain syndrome, characterized by epigastric pain and burning, and postprandial distress syndrome (PDS), characterized by early satiation and postprandial fullness [1]. In spite of initial controversy over whether this subdivision was sufficiently evidence-based and whether it impacts on clinical management, an increasing number of observations are supportive of the subdivision in epigastric pain syndrome and PDS [2].

The pathophysiology underlying FD symptoms remains to be fully elucidated, and a variety of mechanisms have been implicated, including disordered gastrointestinal

Table 1. Published studies on the prevalence of hypersensitivity to gastric distention and the relationship with symptoms in FD

First author	n	Prevalence of hypersensitivity, %	Association with symptoms
Mertz [7]	24	66 (fasting)	no significant association
Rhee [10]	64	50 (fasting)	no significant association
Tack [9]	160	34 (fasting)	associated with severity of epigastric pain, belching, weight loss
Boeckxstaens [8]	44	48 (fasting)	no significant association
Farré [15]	62	45 (fasting)	no significant association
		32 (postprandial)	correlated with severity of postprandial fullness, epigastric pain, nausea and bloating

motor function, visceral hypersensitivity, mucosal immune activation and alterations of the brain-gut axis. Visceral hypersensitivity has emerged as a particularly attractive concept as it readily explains the occurrence of symptoms in the absence of organic findings upon routine examination, and especially as it provides a unifying hypothesis for several major functional gastrointestinal disorders such as IBS and functional heartburn [3].

The Presence of Visceral Hypersensitivity in Functional Dyspepsia

The gold standard in assessing visceral hypersensitivity is the use of a barostat device to register symptom reporting while a hollow visceral organ is being distended by an intraluminal balloon [4]. Relatively few gastric barostat studies have compared FD with healthy controls, but all have confirmed that, as a group, FD patients have lower thresholds for first perception and for discomfort or pain during gastric balloon distention [5–10]. As higher symptom reporting in FD patients occurs while the gastric compliance is similar to that of controls, this indicates the presence of increased visceral sensitivity.

The prevalence of hypersensitivity to gastric distention, defined as perception or discomfort thresholds outside the normal range, varies between studies (table 1) and this is at least in part attributable to the use of different approaches to calculate sensitivity to distention and to determine the range of normality [5–10]. The increase of intraballoon pressure over intraabdominal pressure needed to induce discomfort or pain seems to be the most appropriate expression of sensitivity to gastric distention as it yields a meaningful lower range of normal and it is independent from age and body mass index [9].

The Relevance of Visceral Hypersensitivity in Explaining Functional Dyspepsia Symptoms

In a study of 160 FD patients, hypersensitivity to gastric distention was found in approximately one third, and this was associated with a higher prevalence of postprandial pain, belching and weight loss [9]. However, other, although smaller studies, failed to find an association between the FD symptom complex and the presence of hypersensitivity to gastric distention (table 1).

However, both the site and the physiological context of most gastric balloon distention studies can be questioned. First, these studies are confined to addressing sensitivity of the proximal stomach, as this is the site where the barostat balloon locates when studies are performed in the upright position using an air-filled balloon. A dual balloon study of both antrum and proximal stomach in healthy controls showed that the distal stomach is far less compliant and therefore more sensitive to volume-driven distention [11]. In a dual balloon study in FD, patients were hypersensitive to both antral and fundic distentions, and fundic relaxation in response to antral distention or intestinal nutrient infusions was suppressed in FD [12].

Furthermore, one can question the relevance of fasting perception threshold testing in FD, where symptoms occur predominantly in the postprandial period [13]. In FD, sensitivity to gastric balloon distention is increased during the postprandial period compared to fasting, and showed a better association with the symptom pattern and severity than fasting sensitivity to distention [14, 15]. Moreover, postprandial hypersensitivity to gastric distention in FD patients was associated with the presence of fasting hypersensitivity as well as with impaired accommodation, revealing an integration of both sensory and motor dysfunction in generating FD symptoms [15].

Identity of Mechanoreceptors Involved in Visceral Hypersensitivity

During balloon distention, mechanoreceptors must be activated to initiate, convey, or perceive the distending stimulus. Based on studies in animals, gastrointestinal mechanoreceptors can be conceptualized to be either in series or in parallel to smooth muscle fibers. In animals, in parallel mechanoreceptors respond to stimuli that elongate the viscus, while in series mechanoreceptors respond to stimuli that increase the tension within the viscus wall [16]. Based on comparisons beteen isovolumetric and isobaric gastric balloon distentions, and the influence of agents that contract or relax smooth muscle, it seems that in series mechanoreceptors, responsive to increases in gastric wall tension, mediate gastric mechanosensitivity and hypersensitivity [17–19]. This is further supported by studies where the Laplace formula was used to generate wall tension-driven gastric balloon distentions rather than isobaric or isovolumetric distention, revealing that perception intensity was closely correlated to wall tension independently of intragastric volume or pressure [20].

Nature of Afferent Modalities That Are Upregulated in Visceral Hypersensitivity

Animal studies have shown two distinct types of afferents can transmit mechanical stimuli from the gastrointestinal tract to the brain [21]. Wide dynamic-range afferents have low thresholds and respond proportionally to organ distension from low, non-noxious to noxious distension pressures. Pain-specific afferents are a class of high-threshold afferents that are activated by noxious stimuli. Painful stimuli could be generated through these two afferent pathways: via pain-specific afferents or through multimodal (wide dynamic range) afferent pathways [21, 22].

Analyses of the intensity ratings of pain and non-painful sensations during gastric balloon distension showed no differential activation of sensations at lower or higher levels of distension, in health or hypersensitive FD patients [22]. Hence, it seems that wide-range, low-threshold type mechanosensitive afferents are involved in mediating mechanosensitivity and hypersensitivity of the proximal stomach in man. Furthermore, other modalities than mechanosensitivity are also likely to be involved. Studies showing enhanced sensitivity to duodenal acidification or to capsaicin administration in FD establish that chemosensitivity is also enhanced in these patients [23–25].

Mechanisms Involved in the Generation of Visceral Hypersensitivity in Functional Dyspepsia

A source of long-standing controversy is whether symptoms in FD, and visceral hypersensitivity in particular, arise in the gastrointestinal tract or in the brain. Brain imaging studies have shown that activation of the visceral pain neuromatrix occurs at lower balloon distention levels in FD compared to healthy controls, thereby confirming that the higher intensity reporting at similar distention levels in FD has a neurobiological basis [26, 27]. Furthermore, a number of observations support lack of activation of pain-suppressive pathways during gastric balloon distention in FD [26–29]. The brain activation responses to gastric balloon distention and anticipated balloon distention in FD are influenced by hypersensitivity, anxiety and a history of trauma [28, 29]. These observations support the hypothesis that cognitive-affective processes including anticipation of pain and its associated anxiety interfere with pain modulatory mechanisms in the brain in FD, leading to increased pain sensitivity and symptom levels, thereby arguing in favor of a central mechanism for symptom amplification in FD.

While these findings indicate a central mechanism for symptom generation in FD, there is equally compelling evidence for a contribution of peripheral mechanisms. These include signs of low-grade inflammation in the duodenum [30], altered blood immune cell function [31], increasing levels of circulating gut homing T lymphocytes [32], increased mucosal permeability and altered expression of tight junction molecules in the duodenum [33] in FD.

Therapeutic Implications

It is often assumed that antidepressants decrease visceral hypersensitivity, but in the stomach, there is no convincing evidence that amitriptyline or citalopram decrease sensitivity to gastric distention [34, 35].

The involvement of tension-sensitive mechanoreceptors in symptom generation would argue in favor of therapies that relax (proximal) gastric smooth muscle. Acute studies with the fundus-relaxing agents such as the 5-HT1 agonist sumatriptan and the α_2-adrenergic agonist clonidine provided early proof-of-concept for this hypothesis [19]. More recently, the 5-HT_{1A} agonist buspirone, used as an anxiolytic, was shown to dose-dependently relax the proximal stomach [36], and in controlled studies both 5-HT_{1A} agonists buspirone and tandospirone improved FD symptoms over placebo, and this was not correlated with changes in anxiety or depression ratings [37, 38].

Most recently, acotiamide, a muscarinic autoreceptor antagonist and cholinesterase inhibitor with fundus-relaxing properties [39, 40], was shown to be efficacious in a phase 3 trial in FD/PDS and has been approved for the treatment of FD in Japan [41]. Additional studies in other parts of the world are eagerly awaited.

References

1 Tack J, Talley NJ, Camilleri M, Holtmann G, Hu P, Malagelada JR, Stanghellini V: Functional gastroduodenal disorders. Gastroenterology 2006;130:1466–1479.

2 Tack J, Talley NJ: Functional dyspepsia-symptoms, definitions and validity of the Rome III criteria. Nat Rev Gastroenterol Hepatol 2013;10:134–141.

3 Camilleri M, Coulie B, Tack J: Visceral hypersensitivity: facts, speculations and challenges. Gut 2000; 48:125–131.

4 Whitehead WE, Delvaux M, Azpiroz F, Barlow J, Bradley L, Camilleri M, Crowell MD, Enck P, Fioramonti J, Tack J, Mayer EA, Morteau O, Phillips SF, Thompson DG, Wingate DL: Standardization of procedures for testing smooth muscle tone and sensory thresholds in the gastrointestinal tract. Dig Dis Sci 1997;42:223–241.

5 Bradette M, Pare P, Douville P, Morin A: Visceral perception in health and functional dyspepsia. Crossover study of gastric distensions with placebo and domperidone. Dig Dis Sci 1991;36:52–58.

6 Mearin F, Cucala M, Azpiroz F, Malagelada JR: The origin of symptoms on the brain-gut axis in functional dyspepsia. Gastroenterology 1991;101:999–1006.

7 Mertz H, Fullerton S, Naliboff B, Mayer EA: Symptoms and visceral perception in severe functional and organic dyspepsia. Gut 1998;42:814–822.

8 Boeckxstaens GE, Hirsch DP, Kuiken SD, Heisterkamp SH, Tytgat GN: The proximal stomach and postprandial symptoms in functional dyspeptics. Am J Gastroenterol 2002;97:40–48.

9 Tack J, Caenepeel P, Fischler B, Piessevaux H, Janssens J: Symptoms associated with hypersensitivity to gastric distensions in functional dyspepsia. Gastroenterology 2001;121:526–535.

10 Rhee PL, Kim YH, Son HJ, Kim JJ, Koh KC, Paik SW, Rhee JC, Choi KW: Evaluation of individual symptoms acannot predict presence of gastric hypersensitivity in functional dyspepsia. Dig Dis Sci 2000;45: 1680–1684.
11 Lee KJ, Vos R, Janssens J, Tack J: Differences in the sensorimotor response to distension between the proximal and distal stomach in humans. Gut 2004; 53:938–943.
12 Caldarella MP, Azpiroz F, Malagelada JR: Antrofundic dysfunctions in functional dyspepsia. Gastroenterology 2003;124:1220–1229.
13 Bisschops R, Karamanolis G, Arts J, Caenepeel P, Verbeke K, Janssens J, Tack J: Relationship between symptoms and ingestion of a meal in functional dyspepsia. Gut 2008;57:1495–1503.
14 Thumshirn M, Camilleri M, Saslow SB, Williams DE, Burton DD, Hanson RB: Gastric accommodation in non-ulcer dyspepsia and the roles of *Helicobacter pylori* infection and vagal function. Gut 1999; 44:55–64.
15 Farré R, Vanheel H, Vanuytsel T, Masaoka T, Törnblom H, Simrén M, Van Oudenhove L, Tack J: In functional dyspepsia, hypersensitivity to postprandial distention correlates with meal-related symptom severity. Gastroenterology 2013;145:566–573.
16 Zagorodnyuk VP, Chen BN, Brookes SJ: Intraganglionic laminar endings are mechano-transduction sites of vagal tension receptors in the guinea-pig stomach. J Physiol 2001;534:255–268.
17 Notivol R, Coffin B, Azpiroz F, et al: Gastric tone determines the sensitivity of the stomach to distention. Gastroenterology 1995;108:330–336.
18 Piessevaux H, Tack J, Wilmer A, Coulie B, Geubel A, Janssens J: Perception of changes in wall tension in the proximal stomach in humans. Gut 2001;49:203–208.
19 Tack J, Caenepeel P, Fischler B, Piessevaux H, Janssens J: Role of tension receptors in functional dyspepsia with hypersensitivity to gastric distention. Gastroenterology 2002;127:1058–1066.
20 Distrutti E, Azpiroz F, Soldevilla A, Malagelada J-R: Gastric wall tension determines perception of gastric distention. Gastroenterology 1999;116:1035–1042.
21 Gebhart GF: Pathobiology of visceral pain: molecular mechanisms and therapeutic implications IV. Visceral afferent contributions to the pathobiology of visceral pain. Am J Physiol Gastrointest Liver Physiol 2000;278:G834–G838.
22 Vandenberghe J, Vos R, Persoons P, et al: Dyspeptic patients with visceral hypersensitivity: sensitisation of pain specific or multimodal pathways? Gut 2005; 54:914–919.
23 Samsom M, Verhagen MA, vanBerge Henegouwen GP, Smout AJ: Abnormal clearance of exogenous acid and increased acid sensitivity of the proximal duodenum in dyspeptic patients. Gastroenterology 1999;116:515–520.
24 Lee KJ, Demarchi B, Demedts I, Sifrim D, Raeymaekers P, Tack J: A pilot study on duodenal acid exposure and its relationship to symptoms in functional dyspepsia with prominent nausea. Am J Gastroenterol 2004;99:1765–1773.
25 Hammer J, Führer M, Pipal L, Matiasek J: Hypersensitivity for capsaicin in patients with functional dyspepsia. Neurogastroenterol Motil 2008;20:125–133.
26 Vandenberghe J, Dupont P, Fischler B, Bormans G, Persoons P, Janssens J, Tack J: Regional brain activation during proximal stomach distention in humans: a positron emission tomography study. Gastroenterology 2005;128:564–573.
27 Vandenberghe J, Dupont P, Van Oudenhove L, Bormans G, Demyttenaere K, Fischler B, Geeraerts B, Janssens J, Tack J: Regional cerebral blood flow during gastric balloon distention in functional dyspepsia. Gastroenterology 2007;132:1684–1693.
28 Van Oudenhove L, Vandenberghe J, Dupont P, Geeraerts B, Vos R, Dirix S, Bormans G, Vanderghinste D, Van Laere K, Demyttenaere K, Fischler B, Tack J: Abnormal regional brain activity during rest and (anticipated) gastric distension in functional dyspepsia and the role of anxiety: a H(2)(15)O-PET study. Am J Gastroenterol 2010;105:913–924.
29 Van Oudenhove L, Vandenberghe J, Dupont P, Geeraerts B, Vos R, Dirix S, Van Laere K, Bormans G, Vanderghinste D, Demyttenaere K, Fischler B, Tack J: Regional brain activity in functional dyspepsia: a H(2)(15)O-PET study on the role of gastric sensitivity and abuse history. Gastroenterology 2010; 139:36–47.
30 Kindt S, Van Oudenhove L, Broekaert D, Kasran A, Ceuppens JL, Bossuyt X, Fischler B, Tack J: Immune dysfunction in patients with functional gastrointestinal disorders. Neurogastroenterol Motil 2009;21: 389–398.
31 Kindt S, Tertychnyy A, de Hertogh G, Geboes K, Tack J: Intestinal immune activation in presumed post-infectious functional dyspepsia. Neurogastroenterol Motil 2009;21:832-e56.
32 Liebregts T, Adam B, Bredack C, Gururatsakul M, Pilkington KR, Brierley SM, Blackshaw LA, Gerken G, Talley NJ, Holtmann G: Small bowel homing T cells are associated with symptoms and delayed gastric emptying in functional dyspepsia. Am J Gastroenterol 2011;106:1089–1098.
33 Vanheel H, Vicario M, Vanuytsel T, Van Oudenhove L, Martinez C, Keita AV, Pardon N, Santos J, Söderholm JD, Tack J, Farré R: Impaired duodenal mucosal integrity and low-grade inflammation in functional dyspepsia. Gut 2013, E-pub ahead of print.
34 Mertz H, Fass R, Kodner A, Yan-Go F, Fullerton S, Mayer EA: Effect of amitriptyline on symptoms, sleep, and visceral perception in patients with functional dyspepsia. Am J Gastroenterol 1998;93:160–165.

35 Ladabaum U, Glidden D: Effect of the selective serotonin reuptake inhibitor sertraline on gastric sensitivity and compliance in healthy humans. Neurogastroenterol Motil 2002;14:395–402.
36 Van Oudenhove L, Kindt S, Vos R, Coulie B, Tack J: Influence of buspirone on gastric sensorimotor function in man. Aliment Pharmacol Ther 2008;28: 1326–1333.
37 Tack J, Janssen P, Masaoka T, Farré R, Van Oudenhove L: Efficacy of buspirone, a fundus-relaxing drug, in patients with functional dyspepsia. Clin Gastroenterol Hepatol 2012;10:1239–1245.
38 Miwa H, Nagahara A, Tominaga K, Yokoyama T, Sawada Y, Inoue K, Ashida K, Fukuchi T, Hojo M, Yamashita H, Tomita T, Hori K, Oshima T: Efficacy of the 5-HT1A agonist tandospirone citrate in improving symptoms of patients with functional dyspepsia: a randomized controlled trial. Am J Gastroenterol 2009;104:2779–2787.
39 Tack J, Masclee A, Heading R, Berstad A, Piessevaux H, Popiela T, Vandenberghe A, Kato H: A dose-ranging, placebo-controlled, pilot trial of Acotiamide in patients with functional dyspepsia. Neurogastroenterol Motil 2009;21:272–280.
40 Kusunoki H, Haruma K, Manabe N, Imamura H, Kamada T, Shiotani A, Hata J, Sugioka H, Saito Y, Kato H, Tack J: Therapeutic efficacy of acotiamide in patients with functional dyspepsia based on enhanced postprandial gastric accommodation and emptying: randomized controlled study evaluation by real-time ultrasonography. Neurogastroenterol Motil 2012;24:540–545, e250–e251.
41 Matsueda K, Hongo M, Tack J, Saito Y, Kato H: A placebo-controlled trial of acotiamide for meal-related symptoms of functional dyspepsia. Gut 2012; 61:821–828.

Jan Tack, MD, PhD
TARGID
Herestraat 49
BE–3000 Leuven (Belgium)
E-Mail jan.tack@med.kuleuven.be

Quigley EMM, Hongo M, Fukudo S (eds): Functional and GI Motility Disorders.
Front Gastrointest Res. Basel, Karger, 2014, vol 33, pp 45–54 (DOI: 10.1159/000356739)

Chronic Intestinal Pseudo-Obstruction: A Neuropathological Approach

Roberto De Giorgio[a] • Elisa Boschetti[a, b] • Francesca Bianco[a] • Rosanna F. Cogliandro[a] • Umberto Volta[a] • Giacomo Caio[a] • Roberto Corinaldesi[a] • Vincenzo Stanghellini[a]

Departments of [a]Medical and Surgical Sciences and [b]Biomedical and Neuro-Motor Sciences, University of Bologna, Bologna, Italy

Abstract

Chronic intestinal pseudo-obstruction (CIPO) is a rare syndrome at the extreme end of severe functional bowel disorders. The clinical picture is characterized by a marked impairment of gut propulsive motility, thus mimicking a mechanical obstruction in the absence of any detectable organic cause constricting the gastrointestinal tract. CIPO is still a clinical challenge, and histopathology may be a valuable tool in the diagnostic workup. The histopathological correlates in CIPO include neural, interstitial cells of Cajal (ICC), and/or muscle abnormalities (hence, neuropathy, myopathy and ICC abnormalities), either alone or in combination. Apart from generating a diagnosis, detection of a given histopathological pattern may provide physicians with a guide to prognosis; thus, CIPO patients with an underlying myopathy usually have the poorest outcome compared to those with neuropathy or other patterns. Similar considerations can be applied to genetic forms of CIPO. Peculiar neuropathic/myopathic features, i.e. eosinophilic intraneuronal inclusions in enteric neurons, myenteric/submucosal ganglioneuromas of the enteric nervous system, and a more prominent involvement of the longitudinal rather than the circular layer throughout the gut may suggest CIPO of genetic origin. Another important aspect pertains to the identification of an immune-mediated/inflammatory neuropathy/leiomyositis that can be managed with immunosuppressive drugs. Although still inconclusive, the data published so far are promising and pave the way for future, well-designed trials to test the actual efficacy of immunosuppressive drugs in patients with CIPO due to an underlying inflammatory neuropathy. Future research on gut neuro-ICC-muscular abnormalities is expected to improve diagnostic and therapeutic strategies in patients with CIPO.

Chronic intestinal pseudo-obstruction (CIPO) represents the 'tip of the iceberg' of functional gastrointestinal (GI) disorders. Similarly to any chronic organ failure, CIPO can be viewed as the end result of several abnormalities (either of unknown origin – 'idiopathic' – or secondary to a wide array of pathological conditions) affecting the morphofunctional integrity of the gut neuromuscular layer. Thus, CIPO is characterized by a marked impairment of gut motor coordination/propulsion mimicking a mechanical obstruction in the absence of any demonstrable lesion occluding the gut lumen (thereby 'intestinal pseudo-obstruction', a term introduced by Dudley et al. [1] in the late 1950s). The altered motility in CIPO patients is unavoidably accompanied by changes of other GI functions, i.e. secretion and absorption, which are responsible for nutritional deficits and even, in some cases, overt malnutrition. Thus CIPO is an important cause of chronic intestinal failure and represents ~20% of all adult cases of this syndrome [2, 3]. The small bowel is mainly affected, although any segment of the GI tract may be involved, and clinical manifestations vary during the natural history of this syndrome. In addition, extra-GI manifestations and the extent of malnutrition contribute to the clinical features of CIPO. The actual prevalence and incidence of CIPO remain unknown, while, similarly to other functional GI disorders, females appear to be more prone to this condition [2, 3].

CIPO is a clinical challenge for several reasons: (1) it is rare, hence many physicians, including GI specialists, have limited knowledge about this condition; (2) it is frequently misdiagnosed (i.e. often confused with mechanical causes of intestinal subocclusion responsible for repeated, useless and life-threatening surgical interventions); (3) the clinical picture, being characterized by disabling digestive symptoms between recurrent subocclusive episodes and malnutrition, is often difficult to interpret; (4) life-threatening complications, especially infections causing septicemia, can commonly occur; (5) there are no effective therapeutic options: prokinetic agents, aimed at restoring at least in part gut physiology, have shown limited efficacy. The mainstay of the treatment of patients with CIPO is enteral or, more commonly, parenteral nutrition which is, however, often accompanied by complications (e.g. infections, liver insufficiency). Thus, taking all these issues together, CIPO patients have a poor quality of life, much worse than that of any other functional gut disorders, along with an established mortality rate [3, 4].

The diagnosis of CIPO is mainly supported by clinical features, i.e. symptoms and signs of recurrent subocclusive episodes, associated with radiological evidence of air-fluid levels, with or without bowel dilatation. Furthermore, the diagnostic workup includes a number of noninvasive and invasive tests aimed at ruling out mechanical causes of intestinal subocclusion or providing possible pathophysiological correlates (e.g. neuropathic or myopathic patterns on antroduodenojejunal manometry). Laboratory tests may be useful particularly in secondary forms (e.g. diabetes mellitus, autoimmune disorders and paraneoplastic syndromes) of CIPO. Tissue analysis of biopsy material/surgical specimens may also represent an important aid to the diagnosis [3].

The purpose of this chapter is to review the growing knowledge of the histopathology of CIPO in adult patients, covering several aspects, including the reasons to collect gut full-thickness tissue samples, who should be biopsied and, especially, the results of histopathological examination with possible clinical implications.

Why Tissue Sampling and Which Patients Should Be Biopsied?

The rationale behind collecting gut full-thickness tissue samples is to provide clinicians with a histopathological 'gold-standard' and indicate the possible abnormalities affecting the main control mechanisms regulating gut physiology, i.e. extrinsic and/or intrinsic neurons (also referred to as the enteric nervous system, ENS) supplying the gut; the interstitial cells of Cajal (ICC; the 'pace-makers' of GI motility and regulators of neuromuscular transmission), and enteric smooth muscle (the final effector cells of the gut). The changes affecting these cellular systems are tightly linked to the pathophysiology of the severe dysmotility and may provide indicators, not only towards the correct diagnosis but also towards prognosis and management of patients with CIPO. Only full-thickness specimens have shown the necessary reliability for a thorough histopathological analysis.

In the past, enthusiasm for histopathological analysis of gut full-thickness biopsies obtained from patients with CIPO was often challenged by evidence that traditional surgical approaches worsened the underlying dysmotility and facilitated adhesions. Furthermore, pathologists often discouraged clinicians by reporting an 'apparently normal' neuromuscular layer in cases with marked motor impairment accompanied by frank intestinal dilatation. In recent years, however, impressive technological advances have regenerated the physician's interest in gut full-thickness biopsy in CIPO. Several minimally invasive procedures, including either laparoscopic surgery (or very recently endoscopic approaches, e.g. natural-orifice transluminal endoscopic surgery) have shown a high diagnostic yield and safety [5]. Furthermore, guidelines proposed by the Gastro 2009 International Working Group helped to find consensus about technical aspects (e.g. tissue collection and processing) and histopathological reporting of results in a variety of GI neuromuscular disorders, including CIPO [6, 7].

Should we biopsy all patients with CIPO or some selected cases? Although minimally invasive approaches have limited the risk of surgery, it is useful to define the right candidate who should undergo gut tissue sampling for histopathological analysis. In the absence of clinical guidelines, accumulated experience indicates that the following CIPO patients may be biopsied: (1) idiopathic cases, particularly those with a recent onset likely of postinfectious origin; (2) progressive, rapidly evolving forms refractory to any therapeutic options; (3) patients with severe symptoms (e.g. abdominal pain often refractory to major analgesic drugs) lacking detectable radiologic and endoscopic correlates. In contrast, in CIPO cases with a clear origin (i.e. secondary forms of CIPO), tissue sampling may be less clinically meaningful as many systemic diseases are known to affect the GI neuromuscular layer.

What Are the Results of Histopathology?

There are three main areas of histopathological analysis, i.e. idiopathic, genetic and secondary CIPO. Herein, idiopathic and genetic CIPO will be reviewed, while secondary CIPO lacks systematic analysis based on gut full-thickness biopsy. Nonetheless, two possible exceptions are represented by diabetes mellitus and Parkinson's disease. However, a thorough histopathological evaluation has been performed in clinical phenotypes distinct from CIPO, i.e. gastroparesis and severe constipation. Neuropathological and ICC changes have been detected in the gastric neuromuscular layer of patients with diabetic gastroparesis [8], whereas Lewy body pathology (mainly neurites) was visualized in submucosal neurons of the colon from constipated patients with Parkinson's disease [9]. It is likely that these abnormalities may involve the ENS and ICC more diffusely throughout the gut, but consistent data in CIPO related to diabetes mellitus and Parkinson's disease are still lacking.

Enteric neuropathies, myopathies and, although at a lower level of evidence, ICC abnormalities, may underlie idiopathic CIPO [7].

Neuropathies

From a pathological standpoint, enteric neuropathies can be either degenerative or inflammatory.

Degenerative (noninflammatory) neuropathies are still poorly understood. Some cases may reveal an apparently normal ENS and, therefore, a quantitative analysis of enteric ganglia and neuronal cell bodies would be advisable. However, quantitative analysis of the ENS is a complex and time-consuming approach not readily feasible in routine pathology laboratories. In addition, the lack of normative data in the human ENS contributes to increase the uncertainty experienced by pathologists faced with cases of enteric neuropathies requiring a quantitative analysis. When possible (and based on control values of individual laboratories), quantitative changes in enteric neuropathies may reveal a reduced number of myenteric (more affected than the submucosal) ganglia and ganglion cell bodies, hence the term 'oligoneuronal hypoganglionosis' [10]. As opposed to loss of neurons, a neuropathic pattern may also be identified in conditions characterized by 'giant' enteric ganglia likely due to an increase in the number of neurons (and probably glial cells) as exemplified in some genetic disorders (see below); also, an increased number of ganglion cells has been reported in pediatric cases of CIPO with neuronal intestinal dysplasia type B (not covered in this chapter).

Qualitative findings in degenerative neuropathies include swollen ganglion cell bodies and nerve processes, fragmentation and loss of axons [2, 11–13]. In our hands, qualitative evidence of ENS degeneration has been demonstrated in 10 out of 11 CIPO patients with available histopathology [2]. Neurodegenerative mechanisms in the ENS remain largely undefined and may include factors ranging from altered calcium signaling, mitochondrial dysfunction, to production of free radicals, up to neuronal apoptosis [14]. Abnormalities of enteric glial cells, hence the term 'gliopathy', may also play a role in enteric neuron degeneration, since consistent evidence points to a key role for these cells (once believed to be only supportive elements) in enteric neuron maintenance and survival [15]. However, at the moment the occurrence of a gliopathy represents no more than an interesting possibility which requires confirmatory evidence in CIPO.

Immune-mediated/inflammatory neuropathies can be due to lymphocytes (mainly CD3+ T cells), eosinophils and mast cells infiltrating the ganglionated plexuses of the ENS (hence the term 'enteric ganglionitis'). Commonly, immune/inflammatory cells target primarily myenteric (i.e. 'myenteric ganglionitis') rather than submucosal ganglia as well as axons running throughout the muscular layer of the gut [16]. The definition of lymphocytic ganglionitis is easily applicable when a massive infiltration of lymphocytes can be detected within myenteric ganglia; it is less easily definable in cases with a low-grade infiltrate where a quantitative assessment of the number of lymphocytes may be necessary. The International Working Group on GI neuromuscular disorders proposed that ≥5 lymphocytes/ganglion identify myenteric ganglionitis [7]. Both overt and low-grade lymphocytic myenteric ganglionitis can be detected in CIPO [13, 17–18]. In two independent studies, the histopathological evaluation of intestinal full-thickness biopsies revealed lymphocytic myenteric ganglionitis in 29% [13] and 34% [18] of patients with CIPO. Thus, about 1/3 of patients with CIPO may have an underlying inflammatory (lymphocytic) neuropathy. Lymphocytic myenteric ganglionitis may be associated with neuronal degeneration and loss and even complete ganglion cell depletion ('acquired myenteric aganglionosis') in the most severe cases [17].

Patients with lymphocytic myenteric ganglionitis may develop a humoral response characterized by anti-Hu neuronal antibodies (based on the main molecular target) or referred to as antinuclear neuronal antibodies (ANNA-1) [19]. These autoantibodies have been shown to exert a functional effect since their administration alters the ascending reflex pathway of peristalsis in vitro. Other evidence indicates that anti-Hu antibodies evoke neuronal apoptosis as well as autophagic mechanisms in primary culture of myenteric neurons or neuronal cell lines [20]. Taken together, the lymphocytic infiltrate in myenteric ganglia and anti-neuronal autoantibodies provide a basis to understand the origin of severe dysmotility in patients with an inflammatory neuropathy related to CIPO. Notably, both idiopathic and secondary (paraneoplastic) cases of lymphocytic myenteric ganglionitis share common histopathological features as well as circulating anti-Hu antibodies.

Finally, eosinophils and mast cells infiltrating and/or surrounding myenteric ganglia represent much less common forms of non-lymphocytic ganglionitis in patients with CIPO [21]. These forms of inflammatory neuropathy are characterized by a lower tendency to neurodegeneration compared to lymphocytic myenteric ganglionitis.

Myopathies

Enteric myopathies can be also classified into degenerative and immune-mediated/inflammatory forms.

Cases of familial and sporadic degenerative myopathies have been reported and result in histopathologically similar patterns with both being characterized by smooth muscle cell vacuolization and fibrosis. Familial visceral myopathy (FVM) or 'hollow viscera myopathy' [22] includes two phenotypes, i.e. types I and II. While FVM type I is autosomal dominant and associated with GI (megaesophagus, megaduodenum) and extradigestive (megacystis, mydriasis) manifestations, FVM type II is an autosomal recessive condition coincident with mitochondrial neurogastrointestinal encephalomyopathy (MNGIE) [7]. In sporadic degenerative myopathy, smooth muscle vacuolization and fibrosis involve both circular and longitudinal layers of the gut [7, 11].

Leiomyositis refers to an inflammatory myopathy which can be considered the muscular counterpart of an inflammatory neuropathy. In fact, it is characterized by a lymphocytic infiltrate mainly composed by CD3+ T cells (with both CD4+ and CD8+ subclasses) distributed throughout the two muscular layers and described in particularly severe CIPO [23].

Compared to neuropathies, the prevalence of myopathy in CIPO has been shown to be quite low in most reported series [13, 18], except in one study [12]. In our experience, none of our 11 cases of CIPO showed smooth muscle damage [2]. The immunohistochemical analysis of a panel of molecular targets expressed by the smooth muscle (i.e. smooth muscle myosin heavy chain, smoothelin and histone deacetylase 8) may help the identification of more subtle forms of enteric myopathy in cases with normal smooth muscle α-actin immunolabeling [24].

ICC network abnormalities have been detected in patients with CIPO [25]. In our hands, a decreased ICC density revealed by c-Kit immunohistochemistry has been detected in 49% of CIPO patients [2]. Because ICCs are known key regulator of gut motility [25], their impairment is thought to contribute to gut dysmotility as observed in CIPO. Further studies on ICC abnormalities in CIPO are awaited.

Genetic Chronic Intestinal Pseudo-Obstruction

Most CIPO are sporadic, although different genetic forms, often with a syndromic (multisystemic) phenotype, have been reported [26]. Relatively few histopathological patterns (characterized by either neuropathy or myopathy) are suggestive of a genetic disorder and include: neuronal intranuclear inclusion disease (NIID), multiple endocrine neoplasia type 2B (MEN-2B) and MNGIE.

NIID may be considered a polyglutamine disease characterized by eosinophilic intranuclear inclusions (the hallmark of the disease) in neurons of the central, peripheral and enteric nervous systems along with progressive degeneration and neuronal loss. Molecular analysis indicates that inclusions contain expanded polyglutamine tracts, immunopositive for ubiquitin and, especially, for small ubiquitin-like modifier-1. In cases with predominant autonomic dysfunction, the GI tract involvement features severe dysmotility affecting the esophagus (dysphagia), stomach (gastroparesis) and the whole gut (CIPO). Although most NIID cases are sporadic, occasional instances of familial occurrence indicate a genetic basis, but the responsible gene(s) remains to be identified [27]. NIID overlaps with familial visceral neuropathy, a heterogeneous, poorly defined group of disorders due to abnormalities of the ENS [27].

MEN-2B is a rare autosomal-dominant syndrome characterized by the early development of medullary thyroid cancer in all affected individuals. Pheochromocytomas occur in 50% of patients along with other features, mainly marfanoid habitus, 'blubbery lips' (due to mucosal neuromas), and neuromas of the eyelids [28]. Diffuse ganglioneuromatosis, i.e. transmural 'giant ganglia' with an increased number of neurons and (likely) glial cells of the GI tract occurs in about 40% of patients and is associated with severe constipation/megacolon rather than true CIPO. A specific germline point mutation (methionine to threonine) in *RET* in exon 16 at codon 918 (M918T) occurs in 95% of patients. Other rarer (5%) mutations involve exon 15 at codon 883 (A833F) in the *RET* tyrosine kinase domain [28]. A mutation of *RET* at codon 691 (a glycine to serine conversion) has been identified in a boy with isolated ganglioneuromatosis [29].

In addition to CIPO, patients with MNGIE manifest with cachexia, ptosis, ophthalmoparesis, peripheral neuropathy and white matter changes (leukoencephalopathy) on magnetic resonance imaging of the brain [30]. This syndrome is caused by mutations in the thymidine phosphorylase gene *(TYMP)*. Gut tissue analysis showed that CIPO in patients with MNGIE showed a peculiar histopathological pattern characterized by an underlying enteric myopathy with vacuolization and fibrosis mainly affecting the longitudinal, rather than circular, muscle layer of the small bowel [31].

Are There Clinical Implications of Histopathological Findings?

Despite our understanding of the pathogenetic mechanisms involved in severe GI dysmotility, CIPO is still a clinical challenge. Histopathological analysis and reporting may lend a hand in establishing/confirming the presence of an underlying neuropathy/myopathy/ICC abnormality which, alone or in combination, is responsible for the severe impairment of motility identified in CIPO. This is clinically relevant as pathology still represents a gold standard in medicine [5, 6]. The detection of peculiar features, such as eosinophilic intranuclear inclusions, enteric ganglioneuromatosis and a predominance of longitudinal over circular muscle layer damage, should suggest a genetic form of CIPO and prompt genetic counseling [21].

Prognostic implications may be drawn based on the histopathological picture. Overall, compared to neuropathy, the demonstration of enteric myopathy in CIPO is associated with a worse clinical outcome. Although there are few studies looking at factors influencing the natural history of CIPO, the identification of generalized hypomotility (i.e. a correlate of an underlying myopathy) at intestinal manometry predicts a poor outcome. Also, genetic CIPO usually has a poor prognosis. Finally, the evidence of an immune-mediated/inflammatory neuropathy/myopathy may provide the conceptual basis to target therapy with immunosuppressive drugs. The limited experience acquired so far suggests that, if untreated, immune-mediated neuropathies/leiomyositis may be life-threatening as they evolve towards major neuronal/muscular degeneration leading to severe gut dysfunction [21]. Some studies (mainly case reports or small series) have shown that in a few patients with CIPO and associated inflammatory neuropathy/myopathy, immunosuppressive treatment resulted in significant improvement in severe dysmotility (and related symptoms). However, it must be stressed that: (1) data relied on a limited number of cases; (2) results were completely uncontrolled; (3) doses and type of immunosuppressants varied from case to case. Well-designed, controlled studies are eagerly awaited to prove the efficacy of immunosuppression in inflammatory neuropathy-related CIPO [21]. No evidence is available for other therapeutic options in other forms of neuropathy or ICC abnormality related to CIPO.

Conclusions

CIPO is a rare, disabling syndrome frequently misdiagnosed and associated, overall, with a poor outcome. This chapter reviewed a number of aspects pertinent to gut pathology in patients with CIPO, i.e. why there is a need to perform full-thickness biopsy gut biopsies, who should be biopsied, results of pathological evaluation and, finally, the clinical implications for histopathology. CIPO is still a clinical challenge, and histopathology may represent a valid diagnostic aid by showing neuro-ICC-muscular abnormalities. The histopathological findings can be helpful not only for physicians, but also to guide appropriate information for the patient and the health care system. In particular, the underlying histopathological pattern may have prognostic implications (i.e. patients with genetic and myopathic CIPO usually have the worst clinical outcome). Detection of a peculiar neuropathic/myopathic pattern may suggest a genetic origin. Finally, the evidence of immune-mediated/inflammatory neuropathies/leiomyositis can suggest targeted treatments, i.e. immunosuppressive drugs. While data published so far are promising, more consistent results are eagerly awaited. Ongoing research in GI neuro-ICC-muscular pathology is expected to improve clinical phenotyping, the diagnostic approach and management of patients with CIPO.

Acknowledgements

This work was supported by grants PRIN/COFIN from the Italian Ministry of University, Research and Education 2009 (to R. De G.), and R.F.O. funds from the University of Bologna (R. De G., R.C. and V.S.). R. De G. is the recipient of research grants from 'Fondazione Del Monte di Bologna e Ravenna'.

References

1 Dudley HA, Sinclair IS, McLaren IF, McNair TJ, Newsam JE: Intestinal pseudo-obstruction. J R Coll Surg Edinb 1958;3:206–217.
2 Stanghellini V, Cogliandro RF, De Giorgio R, Barbara G, Morselli-Labate AM, Cogliandro L, Corinaldesi R: Natural history of chronic idiopathic intestinal pseudo-obstruction in adults: a single center study. Clin Gastroenterol Hepatol 2005;3:449–458.
3 De Giorgio R, Cogliandro RF, Barbara G, Corinaldesi R, Stanghellini V: Chronic intestinal pseudo-obstruction: clinical features, diagnosis, and therapy. Gastroenterol Clin North Am 2011;40:787–807.
4 Cogliandro RF, Antonucci A, De Giorgio R, Barbara G, Cremon C, Cogliandro L, Frisoni C, Pezzilli R, Morselli-Labate AM, Corinaldesi R, Stanghellini V: Patient-reported outcomes and gut dysmotility in functional gastrointestinal disorders. Neurogastroenterol Motil 2011;23:1084–1091.
5 Knowles CH, Veress B, Tornblom H, Wallace S, Paraskeva P, Darzi A, Martin JE, Nyberg B, Lindberg G: Safety and diagnostic yield of laparoscopically assisted full-thickness bowel biospy. Neurogastroenterol Motil 2008;20:774–779.
6 Knowles CH, De Giorgio R, Kapur RP, Bruder E, Farrugia G, Geboes K, Gershon MD, Hutson J, Lindberg G, Martin JE, Meier-Ruge WA, Milla PJ, Smith VV, Vandervinden JM, Veress B, Wedel T: Gastrointestinal neuromuscular pathology: guidelines for histological techniques and reporting on behalf of the Gastro 2009 International Working Group. Acta Neuropathol 2009;118:271–301.
7 Knowles CH, De Giorgio R, Kapur RP, Bruder E, Farrugia G, Geboes K, Lindberg G, Martin JE, Meier-Ruge WA, Milla PJ, Smith VV, Vandervinden JM, Veress B, Wedel T: The London Classification of gastrointestinal neuromuscular pathology: report on behalf of the Gastro 2009 International Working Group. Gut 2010;59:882–887.
8 Grover M, Bernard CE, Pasricha PJ, Parkman HP, Abell TL, Nguyen LA, Snape W, Shen KR, Sarr M, Swain J, Kendrick M, Gibbons S, Ordog T, Farrugia G: Platelet-derived growth factor receptor alpha (PDGFRalpha)-expressing 'fibroblast-like cells' in diabetic and idiopathic gastroparesis of humans. Neurogastroenterol Motil 2012;24:844–852.
9 Lebouvier T, Neunlist M, Bruley des Varannes S, Coron E, Drouard A, N'Guyen JM, Chaumette T, Tasselli M, Paillusson S, Flamand M, Galmiche JP, Damier P, Derkinderen P: Colonic biopsies to assess the neuropathology of Parkinson's disease and its relationship with symptoms. PLoS One 2010; 5:e12728.
10 Knowles CH, Veress B, Kapur RP, Wedel T, Farrugia G, Vanderwinden JM, Geboes K, Smith VV, Martin JE, Lindberg G, Milla PJ, De Giorgio R: Quantitation of cellular components of the enteric nervous system in the normal human gastrointestinal tract – report on behalf of the Gastro 2009 International Working Group. Neurogastroenterol Motil 2011;23:115–124.
11 De Giorgio R, Sarnelli G, Corinaldesi R, Stanghellini V: Advances in our understanding of the pathology of chronic intestinal pseudo-obstruction. Gut 2004; 53:1549–1552.
12 Mann SD, Debinski HS, Kamm MA: Clinical characteristics of chronic idiopathic intestinal pseudo-obstruction in adults. Gut 1997;41:675–681.
13 Knowles CH, Silk DB, Darzi A, Veress B, Feakins R, Raimundo AH, Crompton T, Browning EC, Lindberg G, Martin JE: Deranged smooth muscle alpha-actin as a biomarker of intestinal pseudo-obstruction: a controlled multinational case series. Gut 2004;53:1583–1589.
14 De Giorgio R, Camilleri M: Human enteric neuropathies: morphology and molecular pathology. Neurogastroenterol Motil 2004;16:515–531.

15 De Giorgio R, Giancola F, Boschetti E, Abdo H, Lardeux B, Neunlist M: Enteric glia and neuroprotection: basic and clinical aspects. Am J Physiol Gastrointest Liver Physiol 2012;303:G887–G893.
16 De Giorgio R, Guerrini S, Barbara G, Stanghellini V, De Ponti F, Corinaldesi R, Moses PL, Sharkey KA, Mawe GM: Inflammatory neuropathies of the enteric nervous system. Gastroenterology 2004;126:1872–1883.
17 De Giorgio R, Barbara G, Stanghellini V, De Ponti F, Salvioli B, Tonini M, Velio P, Bassotti G, Corinaldesi R: Clinical and morphofunctional features of idiopathic myenteric ganglionitis underlying severe intestinal motor dysfunction: a study of three cases. Am J Gastroenterol 2002;97:2454–2459.
18 Lindberg G, Tornblom H, Iwarzon M, Nyberg B, Martin JE, Veress B: Full-thickness biopsy findings in chronic intestinal pseudo-obstruction and enteric dysmotility. Gut 2009;58:1084–1090.
19 De Giorgio R, Bovara M, Barbara G, Canossa M, Sarnelli G, De Ponti F, Stanghellini V, Tonini M, Cappello S, Pagnotta E, Nobile-Orazio E, Corinaldesi R: Anti-HuD-induced neuronal apoptosis underlying paraneoplastic gut dysmotility. Gastroenterology 2003;125:70–79.
20 Hubball A, Martin JE, Lang B, De Giorgio R, Knowles CH: The role of humoral autoimmunity in gastrointestinal neuromuscular diseases. Prog Neurobiol 2009;87:10–20.
21 Knowles CH, Lindberg G, Panza E, De Giorgio R: New perspectives in the diagnosis and management of enteric neuropathies. Nat Rev Gastroenterol Hepatol 2013;10:206–218.
22 Smith JA, Hauser SC, Madara JL: Hollow visceral myopathy: a light- and electron-microscopic study. Am J Surg Pathol 1982;6:269–275.
23 Dewit S, de Hertogh G, Geboes K, Tack J: Chronic intestinal pseudo-obstruction caused by an intestinal inflammatory myopathy: case report and review of the literature. Neurogastroenterol Motil 2008;20:343–348.
24 Wedel T, Van Eys GJ, Waltregny D, Glenisson W, Castronovo V, Vanderwinden JM: Novel smooth muscle markers reveal abnormalities of the intestinal musculature in severe colorectal motility disorders. Neurogastroenterol Motil 2006;18:526–538.
25 Farrugia G: Interstitial cells of Cajal in health and disease. Neurogastroenterol Motil 2008;20(suppl 1):54–63.
26 Panza E, Knowles CH, Graziano C, Thapar N, Burns AJ, Seri M, Stanghellini V, De Giorgio R: Genetics of human enteric neuropathies. Prog Neurobiol 2012;96:176–189.
27 Kimber TE, Blumbergs PC, Rice JP, Hallpike JF, Edis R, Thompson PD, Suthers G: Familial neuronal intranuclear inclusion disease with ubiquitin positive inclusions. J Neurol Sci 1998;160:33–40.
28 Raue F, Frank-Raue K: Update multiple endocrine neoplasia type 2. Fam Cancer 2010;9:449–457.
29 Nguyen AT, Zacharin MR, Smith M, Hardikar W: Isolated intestinal ganglioneuromatosis with a new mutation of RET proto-oncogene. Eur J Gastroenterol Hepatol 2006;18:803–805.
30 Garone C, Tadesse S, Hirano M: Clinical and genetic spectrum of mitochondrial neurogastrointestinal encephalomyopathy. Brain 2011;134:3326–3332.
31 Giordano C, Sebastiani M, De Giorgio R, Travaglini C, Tancredi A, Valentino ML, Bellan M, Cossarizza A, Hirano M, d'Amati G, Carelli V: Gastrointestinal dysmotility in mitochondrial neurogastrointestinal encephalomyopathy is caused by mitochondrial DNA depletion. Am J Pathol 2008;173:1120–1128.

Roberto De Giorgio, MD, PhD, AGAF
Department of Clinical Medicine, Building #5 (Nuove Patologie), St. Orsola-Malpighi Hospital
Via Massarenti, 9
IT–40138 Bologna (Italy)
E-Mail roberto.degiorgio@unibo.it

Quigley EMM, Hongo M, Fukudo S (eds): Functional and GI Motility Disorders.
Front Gastrointest Res. Basel, Karger, 2014, vol 33, pp 55–64 (DOI: 10.1159/000356743)

Small Intestinal Dysmotility, Its Role in Irritable Bowel Syndrome and Small Intestinal Bacterial Overgrowth: Assessment and Management

Eamonn M.M. Quigley
Division of Gastroenterology, The Methodist Hospital, Houston, Tex., USA

Abstract

Irritable bowel syndrome (IBS) is one of the most common functional gastrointestinal disorders and, for some sufferers, results in significant impairment in quality of life. From the outset, IBS was regarded as a disorder of gastrointestinal motility, and terms such as 'spastic colon' or even 'spastic colitis' applied. As these terms imply, the focus in the early days of the investigation of the pathophysiology of IBS was on the colon and on the left colon, in particular. Subsequently, as advances in manometric technology permitted reliable recordings of motor activity from the small intestine, alterations in small intestinal motility were described in IBS, at rest, following food ingestion and in response to stressful stimuli; some of the abnormal patterns identified seemed to correlate temporally with certain symptoms. More recently, interest in the potential roles of such phenomena as dysbiosis, low-grade inflammation and enhanced intestinal permeability have renewed interest in the potential role of the small intestine and its neuromuscular apparatus in IBS. Relationships between small intestinal dysmotility and small intestinal bacterial overgrowth (SIBO) are more clear-cut given that impaired gut motor activity is one of the primary factors that predisposes to SIBO. Dysmotility is, indeed, the process underlying the development of SIBO in relation to conditions as diverse as scleroderma, diabetes, and intestinal pseudo-obstruction.

Small Intestinal Motility and the Irritable Bowel Syndrome

Irritable Bowel Syndrome: Definition and Pathophysiology

There is no pathological or biochemical definition of irritable bowel syndrome (IBS); this remains entirely clinical and is based either on the recognition of a symptom complex considered diagnostic, or by the exclusion of other diagnostic possibilities. To promote standardization in clinical research as well as permit a 'positive' clinical diagnosis, various criteria or diagnostic systems have been advanced to facilitate the definition of IBS without recourse to extensive investigations. Of the various schemas that have been proposed, those emanating from the Rome process have been most widely accepted and now form the basis for the definition of subjects in clinical studies in IBS. According to Rome III [1], the most recent iteration of this process, IBS is defined as follows:

Recurrent abdominal pain or discomfort at least 3 days/month in the last 3 months associated with *two or more* of the following:

- Improvement with defecation
- Onset associated with a change in frequency of stool
- Onset associated with a change in form (appearance) of stool

This criterion should be fulfilled for the last 3 months with symptom onset at least 6 months prior to diagnosis.

IBS is, perhaps, the most common and best characterized of a group of disorders that absent any biomarker and well-defined pathophysiology are rather unsatisfactorily described as 'functional'. Included within this term are such disorders as noncardiac chest pain, functional heartburn, functional (or nonulcer) dyspepsia and chronic idiopathic (or functional) constipation. These disorders commonly overlap and share similar demographics and many putative pathophysiological features. For example, these common functional disorders have each been characterized by the presence of variable motor abnormalities and visceral hypersensitivity, as well as of other phenomena, such as autonomic dysfunction, altered central perception of visceral events, hypothalamic-pituitary axis dysfunction, subtle inflammation, alterations in the gut microbiome and a significant role for stress and psychological factors [2]. Another important issue in any consideration of the pathophysiology of IBS is its fluctuating nature. The typical IBS patient reports episodes of intense symptoms separated by periods of well-being; for example, one study documented that IBS patients suffered symptoms on an average of 7 days or 14 h per month [3]. If a motor abnormality is linked to symptoms, the timing of a study, becomes critical; to confuse matters further, symptom expression may vary within the same patient from diarrhea, on one occasion, to constipation, on another; each of these symptoms being associated with quite different motor changes [4, 5].

While the pathophysiology of the IBS remains unclear, several factors have been proposed [6, 7]. It is fair to state that, at this time, the primacy of any one of these factors has not been established in IBS. It remains entirely plausible to propose that a given factor may predominate in an individual patient or that a number may converge to induce symptoms; so far, attempts to associate symptom pattern with pathophysiology have, in general, proven unsuccessful.

Gastrointestinal Motor Dysfunction in Irritable Bowel Syndrome

Dysmotility has long been considered a major factor in the pathophysiology of IBS, as indicated by the use of such terms as the 'spastic colon' or even 'spastic colitis' to describe what is now referred to as IBS. Accordingly, it was suggested that gut spasm or other abnormal contractile activities led to the development of symptoms in IBS, and the gut neuromuscular apparatus continues to be a target for drug development [8]. There are, indeed, several reports of abnormal motor patterns in many parts of the gastrointestinal tract in IBS [9, 10].

Initially, the focus was on the colon, and several electromyographic and manometric abnormalities were described in early studies. IBS patients seemed particularly predisposed to developing colonic dysmotility, often associated with symptoms, in response to food ingestion and on exposure to stressful stimuli. Recent reviews of the literature suggest that there is not good evidence for an abnormality in baseline motor activity in the colon in IBS and that many of the 'abnormalities' described may have been related either to associated psychopathology or to the nonspecific effects of associated constipation or diarrhea [9, 11]. With regard to the latter, it is evident that colonic [12–15] and rectal [16] motor changes, in IBS, may reflect those associated with the predominant symptom, be it diarrhea or constipation, in a given IBS subgroup. These observations are important in that they highlight the ever-present cloud of epiphenomenology that looms over all studies of IBS pathophysiology. The interpretation of such studies is also complicated by our relatively primitive understanding of normal colonic motility as well as its intrinsic variability and sensitivity to extrinsic influences.

Small Intestinal Dysmotility in Irritable Bowel Syndrome

More recently, the emphasis has shifted to the small intestine, not only in terms of motility, but also with regard to such parameters as intestinal permeability and secretion as well as changes in the microbiome and low-grade inflammation. With advances in manometric technology, reliable recordings of small intestinal motor patterns became possible and the description of a number of motor abnormalities in IBS generated considerable interest [10, 17]. While most studies of small intestinal motor activity failed to demonstrate any basic abnormality of the migrating motor complex in IBS [18], a number of studies have revealed a prominence of repetitive bursts of contractions or 'clusters' [18–20]. Indeed, in some of these studies, the appearance of clusters in the jejunum was accompanied by the onset of the patient's typical symptoms [18, 20]. 'Clusters' are not diagnostic of IBS; they are a feature of a wide variety of motor disorders [10, 17]. Furthermore, several other investigators have failed to demonstrate an increased prevalence of 'clusters' among their IBS patients [18–25]. Other abnormalities of small intestinal motor function have been described in IBS, including prominent high-amplitude waves in the terminal ileum and an exaggerated jejunal motor response to meal ingestion [18, 19]. Whether the presence of clusters and other motor abnormalities, in some IBS patients, reflects the effects of associated diarrhea, an undue sensitivity to external stress or, indeed, a basic abnormality of the enteric neuromuscular apparatus remains unresolved. It remains entirely possible that a small number of so-called IBS patients are in reality a part of the spectrum of chronic idiopathic intestinal pseudo-obstruction (CIIP) [17]. In support of this concept are reports of motor abnormalities, in some IBS patients, reminiscent of CIIP and the description of histological abnormalities in the enteric nervous system of the small intestine in a small number of patients with what was described as severe IBS [26].

Though less studied, disturbances in transit have also been demonstrated in IBS. Here again, results are influenced by the nature of the predominant bowel habit [11].

Abnormal Gas Handling: A Unique Motor Abnormality in Irritable Bowel Syndrome

Bloating and distension, sensations typically attributed to 'gas' by IBS sufferers are extremely common, distressful and notoriously difficult to treat in IBS. Despite commonly held beliefs to the contrary, the actual production of gas in the intestine and total intra-abdominal gas volumes have generally been shown to be normal in IBS [27, 28]. How does one then explain a symptom such as distension which has been shown to be real and not imaginary [29]? Of particular interest are observations on the handling of gas by the intestine in IBS [30–32] which suggest that there may be a specific motor disorder in IBS which delays gas transit through the small intestine and leads to gas trapping in intestinal segments. Thus, whereas gas infused into the small intestine was rapidly evacuated through the gut in normal volunteers, a similar infusion resulted in gas retention, symptoms and an increase in abdominal girth in IBS patients [30]. All were reversible by parenteral administration of a prokinetic agent [32], supporting a fundamental role for motility [33, 34]. In normal volunteers, similar sensations can be induced by the voluntary retention of gas [32]. Other factors such as visceral sensation [35], abnormal afferent responses [36] and diaphragmatic and abdominal wall reflexes [37] are also important to the pathogenesis of these common symptoms.

It should be noted that, in contrast to the above studies demonstrating impaired transit of gas, others have reported accelerated transit of a mixed solid-liquid meal in 'bloated' IBS subjects [38]. Motor abnormalities have also been described in the esophagus and stomach in IBS; as evidenced by studies of gastric emptying in patients with IBS and functional dyspepsia, it is clear that many of these reports reflect overlap between IBS and other functional disorders.

Small Intestinal Bacterial Overgrowth in Irritable Bowel Syndrome: Evidence of a Motility Disorder?

More recently, the role of the gut flora in IBS has been taken a stage further with the suggestion that some IBS patients may harbor quantitative changes in the indigenous flora in the small intestine: small intestinal bacterial overgrowth (SIBO) [39–43]. Furthermore, the occurrence of SIBO has been associated with abnormalities in small intestinal motor function [44] and its eradication with symptomatic relief [39, 40]. These striking results have been the target of much criticism on several grounds [45–48]. First, IBS symptoms are nonspecific and may be mimicked by SIBO, regardless of etiology; patient selection is therefore an issue. Second, the hydrogen breath test, which has been the test most widely used to make the diagnosis of SIBO in this context, is subject to considerable error, especially in relation to altered small bowel transit [49]. Third, the prevalence of SIBO has varied according to the criteria used to define a positive test [50]. Fourth, SIBO may be an incidental consequence of a therapeutic agent commonly used in IBS, namely, a proton pump inhibitor [51], and, finally, others have failed to confirm these findings [49, 52–54].

Nevertheless, antibiotic therapy does seem to have some benefits in IBS. Initial studies with neomycin suggested promise [39, 40], and more recent studies employing the nonabsorbable antibiotic, rifaximin, have sustained this promise [55, 56] by demonstrating a durable response (lasting at least up to 12 weeks) following a 10- to 14-day course of rifaximin therapy. However, the eradication of SIBO may not be the sole explanation for the observed responses; indeed, none of the pivotal studies have provided any results of breath tests or jejunal cultures in their IBS populations, rendering correlations between clinical response and SIBO prevalence or eradication purely speculative.

Small Intestinal Motility in Irritable Bowel Syndrome: What Is Its Real Role?

What is the clinical significance of disturbed motor function in IBS? Firstly, it seems reasonable to state that some IBS patients will demonstrate disturbances of colonic or small intestinal motor function, if appropriately studied and, especially, if tested in response to such stimuli as food ingestion and stress. Secondly, it remains difficult to interpret the significance of these findings due to the possible confounding effects of selection bias and such epiphenomena as stress and psychopathology. However, the possibility of a fundamental abnormality of enteric neuromuscular function in some IBS patients cannot be discounted, but is likely to afflict only a minority. Thirdly, changes in motor function could reflect the impact of any one of a number of factors that latterly have been proposed as relevant to IBS: low-grade inflammation, dysbiosis, food intolerance or impaired bile acid absorption [6, 7, 57]. Finally, regardless of the relevance of dysmotility to the fundamental pathogenesis of IBS, its role in symptom generation continues to be supported by the reported efficacy of some antispasmodic drugs in this disorder [58]. It can also be argued that the failure of such agents to provide anything other than transient symptomatic relief during acute 'flares' speaks against the primacy of dysmotility in the pathogenesis of IBS.

Small Intestinal Motility and Small Intestinal Bacterial Overgrowth

Definition

Two potential clinical manifestations of SIBO may be distinguished: (1) SIBO as a cause of maldigestion/malabsorption; here, the clinical presentation can be related to effects of the contaminating organism on host morphology or function which, in turn, result in the clinical consequences typically associated with SIBO, such as steatorrhea, diarrhea, protein-losing enteropathy and/or specific deficiency states. (2) SIBO associated with symptoms or clinical entities in the absence of evidence of maldigestion/malabsorption (e.g. SIBO in association with IBS) and where the pathophysiological linkage with SIBO is less clearly defined.

In relation to the first of these clinical contexts, SIBO can be defined as 'clinical and/or laboratory evidence of maldigestion/malabsorption related to qualitative and/or quantitative alterations in the small intestinal microbiota'. Here, the emphasis is on the clinical context and SIBO is incriminated, firstly, by documenting its presence, and, secondly, by demonstrating a clinical response to its eradication. Here we are dealing with what could be regarded as 'classical' SIBO.

The second scenario, the 'expanded' version of SIBO, has proven much more problematic as much of the evidence advanced to support an association between SIBO and a given entity has been reliant on the performance characteristics of the test used to define it and, specifically, on the ability of that test to distinguish health from disease. Typically, a response to SIBO eradication has not been reported or, if it has, its interpretation remains rather murky. Absent such evidence and lacking biochemical and/or pathological findings that can be plausibly linked to SIBO, it has often been unclear in these situations whether SIBO is a cause, a consequence or an epiphenomenon in relation to the other supposedly associated disorder. The relationship between IBS and SIBO had already been addressed in the preceding section.

Dysmotility and Small Intestinal Bacterial Overgrowth

In health, the most important defensive factors against the development of SIBO are gastric acid and intestinal motor activity. In the stomach, acid kills and suppresses the growth of most organisms that enter from the oropharynx. In the small bowel, the cleansing action of propulsive forces and, especially, phase III of the interdigestive migrating motor complex, limits the ability of bacteria to colonize the small intestine [59]. Accordingly, diseases resulting in impaired intestinal motility are likely to have SIBO as a complication, and virtually every condition that has been linked to small intestinal dysmotility has been associated with SIBO [60–68]. Diabetic autonomic neuropathy and scleroderma are prominent examples of dysmotility-related SIBO. In a patient with diabetes with diarrhea, and, especially in the individual with long-standing type I diabetes [60], SIBO should be sought as a potentially remediable cause. SIBO is common in scleroderma being documented in 43–56% of patients in two recent studies [67, 68]. The prevalence of SIBO in scleroderma has been linked with a higher global symptom score and, especially, among those with a high score for digestive symptoms. Other factors predictive of SIBO, in scleroderma, include the presence of diarrhea and constipation. Eradication of SIBO, successful in 52–73%, results in symptom improvement [67, 68]. Intestinal pseudo-obstruction and jejunal diverticulosis are two less common examples of SIBO based on myogenic or neurogenic intestinal dysmotility. Morphological studies suggest that disorders of intestinal motility such as progressive systemic sclerosis, visceral myopathies and neuropathies play an important role in the formation of small bowel diverticula [69]. Diverticula in the jejunum occur in 0.07–2% of the population and tend to be large and multiple, whereas those in the ileum are small and single. These features explain the observation that symptoms and complications, such as SIBO, have been reported more frequently in association with jejunal than with ileal diverticula. Jejunal diverticula are twice as frequent in men and are observed predominantly among those over 60 years of age.

The relationship between SIBO and impaired motility is clear in the aforementioned disorders; the extent to which dysmotility may contribute to the development of SIBO in other scenarios such as Crohn's disease, celiac disease, cystic fibrosis or liver disease has not be quantitated, but a role is certainly plausible.

References

1 Longstreth GF, Thompson WG, Chey WD, et al: Functional bowel disorders. Gastroenterology 2006; 130:1480–1491.

2 American Gastroenterological Association: Medical position statement: irritable bowel syndrome. Gastroenterology 1997;112:2118–2119.

3 Hungin APS, Tack J, Whorwell PJ, Mearin F: Symptoms and patterns in irritable bowel syndrome in the general population: the truth in IBS (T-IBS) survey. J Gastroenterol Hepatol 2002; 17(suppl):A31.

4 Garrigues V, Mearin F, Badía X, Balboa A, Benavent J, Caballero A, Domínguez E, Díaz-Rubio M, Roset M, Figueras M, Cucala M, RITMO GROUP: Change over time of bowel habit in irritable bowel syndrome: a prospective, observational, 1-year follow-up study (RITMO study). Aliment Pharmacol Ther 2007;25: 323–332.

5 Palsson OS, Baggish JS, Turner MJ, Whitehead WE: IBS patients show frequent fluctuations between loose/watery and hard/lumpy stools: implications for treatment. Am J Gastroenterol 2012;107:286–295.

6 Camilleri M: Peripheral mechanisms in irritable bowel syndrome. New Engl J Med 2012;367:1626–1635.

7 Quigley EM: Bugs on the brain; brain in the gut – seeking explanations for common gastrointestinal symptoms. Ir J Med Sci 2013;182:1–6.
8 McKee DP, Quigley EMM: Intestinal motility in irritable bowel syndrome: is IBS a motility disorder? 1. Definition of IBS and colonic motility. Dig Dis Sci 1993;38:1761–1772.
9 De Ponti F: Drug development for the irritable bowel syndrome: current challenges and future perspectives. Front Pharmacol 2013;4:1–12.
10 McKee DP, Quigley EMM: Intestinal motility in irritable bowel syndrome: is IBS a motility disorder? 2. Motility of the small bowel, esophagus, stomach and gall bladder. Dig Dis Sci 1993;38: 1763–1782.
11 Kellow JE, Azpiroz F, Delvaux M, Gebhart GF, Mertz HR, Quigley EM, Smout AJ: Applied principles of neurogastroenterology: physiology/motility sensation. Gastroenterology 2006;130:1412–1420.
12 Bassotti G, Chistolini F, Marinozzi G, Morelli A: Abnormal colonic propagated activity in patients with slow transit constipation and constipation predominant irritable bowel syndrome. Digestion 2003;68: 178–183.
13 Clemens CH, Samsom M, Van Berge Henegouwen GP, Smout AJ: Abnormalities of left colonic motility in ambulant non-constipated patients with irritable bowel syndrome. Dig Dis Sci 2003;48:74–82.
14 Steens J, van der Schaar PJ, Denning C, Brussee J, Masclee AA: Compliance, tone and sensitivity of the rectum in different subtypes of irritable bowel syndrome. Neurogastroenterol Motil 2002;14:241–247.
15 Cole SJ, Duncan HD, Claydon AH, Austin D, Bowling TE, Silk DB: Distal colonic motor activity in four subgroups of patients with irritable bowel syndrome. Dig Dis Sci 2002;47:345–355.
16 Distrutti E, Savioli B, Azpiroz F, Malagelada J-R: Rectal function and bowel habit in irritable bowel syndrome. Am J Gastroenterol 2004;99:131–137.
17 Quigley EMM: Disturbances in small bowel motility. Baillieres Best Pract Res Clin Gastroenterol 1999;13: 385–395.
18 Kellow JE, Phillips SF: Altered small bowel motility in irritable bowel syndrome is correlated with symptoms. Gastroenterology 1987;92:1885–1893.
19 Kellow JE, Miller LJ, Phillips SF, Zinsmeister AR: Dysmotility of the small intestine in irritable bowel syndrome. Gut 1988;29:1236–1243.
20 Kellow JE, Gill RC, Wingate DL: Prolonged ambulant recordings of small bowel motility demonstrate abnormalities in the irritable bowel syndrome. Gastroenterology 1990;98:1208–1218.
21 Gorard DA, Libby GW, Farthing MJ: Ambulatory small bowel motility in 'diarrhoea' predominant irritable syndrome. Gut 1994;35:203–210.
22 Quigley EMM, Donovan JP, Lane MJ, Gallagher TF: Antroduodenal manometry – usefulness and limitations as an outpatient study. Dig Dis Sci 1992;37:20–28.
23 Schmidt T, Hackelsberger N, Widmer R, Meisel C, Pfeiffer A, Kaess H: Ambulatory 24-hour jejunal motility in diarrhea-predominant irritable bowel syndrome. Scand J Gastroenterol 1996;31:581–589.
24 Small PK, Loudon MA, Hau CM, Noor N, Campbell FC: Large-scale ambulatory study of post-prandial jejunal motility in irritable bowel syndrome. Scand J Gastroenterol 1997;32:39–47.
25 Gorard DA, Vesselinova-Jenkins CK, Libby GW, Farthing MJ: Migrating motor complex in sleep in health and irritable bowel syndrome. Dig Dis Sci 1995;40:2383–2389.
26 Tornblom H, Lindberg G, Nyberg B, Veress B: Full-thickness biopsy of the jejunum reveals inflammation and enteric neuropathy in irritable bowel syndrome. Gastroenterology 2002;123:1972–1979.
27 Lasser RB, Bond JH, Levitt MD: Role of intestinal gas in functional abdominal pain. N Engl J Med 1975; 293:524–526.
28 Mc Williams SR, Mc Laughlin PD, O'Connor OJ, Desmond AN, Ní Laoíre A, Shanahan F, Quigley EM, Maher MM: Computed tomography assessment of intestinal gas volumes in functional gastrointestinal disorders. J Neurogastroenterol Motil 2012;18:419–425.
29 Lewis MJV, Reilly B, Houghton LA, Whorwell PJ: Ambulatory abdominal wall plethysmography: towards objective assessment of abdominal distension in irritable bowel syndrome. Gut 2001;48:216–220.
30 Serra J, Azpiroz F, Malagelada J-R: Impaired transit and tolerance of intestinal gas in the irritable bowel syndrome. Gut 2001;48:14–19.
31 Serra J, Salvioli B, Azpiroz F, Malagelada JR: Lipid-induced intestinal gas retention in irritable bowel syndrome. Gastroenterology 2002;123:700–706.
32 Caldarella M-P, Serra J, Azpiroz F, Malagelada J-R: Prokinetc effects in patients with intestinal gas retention. Gastroenterology 2002;122:1748–1755.
33 Serra J, Azpiroz F, Malagelada J-R: Mechanisms of intestinal gas retention in humans: impaired propulsion versus obstructed evacuation. Am J Physiol 2001;281:G138–G150.
34 Serra J, Villoria A, Azpiroz F, Lobo B, Santos J, Accarino A, Malgelada J-R: Impaired intestinal gas propulsion in manometrically proven dysmotility and in irritable bowel syndrome. Neurogastroenterol Motil 2010;22:401–406, e91–e92.
35 Galati JS, McKee DP, Quigley EMM: The response to intraluminal gas in the irritable bowel syndrome: motility versus perception. Dig Dis Sci 1995;40: 1381–1387.

36 Accarino AM, Azpiroz F, Malagelada J-R: Selective dysfunction of mechanosensitive afferents in the irritable bowel syndrome. Gastroenterology 1995;108: 636–643.

37 Accarino A, Perez F, Azpiroz F, Quiroga S, Malagelada JR: Abdominal distention results from caudo-ventral redistribution of contents. Gastroenterology 2009;136:1544–1551.

38 Hebden JM, Blackshaw E, D'Amato M, Perkins AC, Spiller RC: Abnormalities of GI transit in bloated irritable bowel syndrome: effect of bran on transit and symptoms. Am J Gastroenterol 2002;97:2315–2320.

39 Pimentel M, Chow EJ, Lin HC: Eradication of small intestinal bacterial overgrowth reduces symptoms of irritable bowel syndrome. Am J Gastroenterol 2000; 95:3503–3506.

40 Pimentel M, Chow EJ, Lin HC: Normalization of lactulose breath testing correlates with symptom improvement in irritable bowel syndrome. A double-blind, randomized, placebo-controlled study. Am J Gastroenterol 2003;98:412–419.

41 Nucera G, Gabrielli M, Lupascu A, Lauritano EC, Santoliquido A, Cremonini F, Cammarota G, Tondi P, Pola P, Gasbarrini G, Gasbarrini A: Abnormal breath tests to lactose, fructose and sorbitol in irritable bowel syndrome may be explained by small intestinal bacterial overgrowth. Aliment Pharmacol Ther 2005;21:1391–1395.

42 Lupascu A, Gabrielli M, Lauritano EC, Scarpellini E, Santoliquido A, Cammarota G, Flore R, Tondi P, Pola P, Gasbarrini G, Gasbarrini A: Hydrogen glucose breath test to detect small intestinal bacterial overgrowth: a prevalence case-control study in irritable bowel syndrome. Aliment Pharmacol Ther 2005;22:1157–1160.

43 Ghoshal UC, Kumar S, Mehrotra M, Lakshmi C, Misra A: Frequency of small intestinal bacterial overgrowth in patients with irritable bowel syndrome and chronic non-specific diarrhea. J Neurogastroenterol Motil 2010;16:40–46.

44 Pimentel M, Soffer EE, Chow EJ, Kong Y, Lin HC: Lower frequency of MMC is found in IBS subjects with abnormal lactulose breath test, suggesting bacterial overgrowth. Dig Dis Sci 2002;47:2639–2643.

45 Hasler WL: Lactulose breath testing, bacterial overgrowth, and IBS: just a lot of hot air? Gastroenterology 2003;125:1898–1900.

46 Quigley EM: A 51-year-old with irritable bowel syndrome: test or treat for bacterial overgrowth? Clin Gastroenterol Hepatol 2007;5:1140–1143.

47 Vanner S: The lactulose breath test for diagnosing SIBO in IBS patients: another nail in the coffin. Am J Gastroenterol 2008;103:964–965.

48 Vanner S: The small intestinal bacterial overgrowth Irritable bowel syndrome hypothesis: implications for treatment. Gut 2008;57:1315–1321.

49 Yu D, Cheesman F, Vanner S: Combined oro-cecal scintigraphy and lactulose hydrogen breath testing demonstrate that breath testing detects oro-cecal transit, not small intestinal bacterial overgrowth in patients with IBS. Gut 2011;60:334–340.

50 Ford AC, Spiegel BM, Talley NJ, Moayyedi P: Small intestinal bacterial overgrowth in irritable bowel syndrome: systematic review and meta-analysis. Clin Gastroenterol Hepatol 2009;7:1279–1286.

51 Spiegel BM, Chey WD, Chang L: Bacterial overgrowth and irritable bowel syndrome: unifying hypothesis or a spurious consequence of proton pump inhibitors? Am J Gastroenterol 2008;103:2972–2976.

52 Walters B, Vanner SJ: Detection of bacterial overgrowth in IBS using the lactulose H2 breath test: comparison with 14C-D-xylose and healthy controls. Am J Gastroenterol 2005;100:1566–1570.

53 Posserud ISP, Bjornsson ES, Abrahamsson H, Simren M: Small intestinal bacterial overgrowth in patients with irritable bowel syndrome. Gut 2007;56: 802–808.

54 Bratten JR, Spanier J, Jones MP: Lactulose breath testing does not discriminate patients with irritable bowel syndrome from healthy controls. Am J Gastroenterol 2008;103:958–963.

55 Pimentel M, Park S, Mirocha J, Kane SV, et al: The effect of a nonabsorbed oral antibiotic (rifaximin) on the symptoms of the irritable bowel syndrome: a randomized trial. Ann Intern Med 2006;145:557–563.

56 Pimentel M, Lembo A, Chey WD, Zakko S, Ringel Y, Yu J, Mareya SM, Shaw AL, Bortey E, Forbes WP, TARGET Study Group: Rifaximin therapy for patients with irritable bowel syndrome without constipation. N Engl J Med 2011;364:22–32.

57 Hughes PA, Zola H, Penttila IA, Blackshaw LA, Andrews JM, Krumbiegel D: Immune activation in irritable bowel syndrome: can neuroimmune interactions explain symptoms? Am J Gastroenterol 2013; 108:1066–1074.

58 Ford AC, Talley NJ, Spiegel BM, Foxx-Orenstein AE, Schiller L, Quigley EM, Moayyedi P: Effect of fibre, antispasmodics, and peppermint oil in the treatment of irritable bowel syndrome: systematic review and meta-analysis. BMJ 2008;337:a2313.

59 Vantrappen G, Janssens J, Hellemans J, Ghoos Y: The interdigestive motor complex of normal subjects and patients with bacterial overgrowth of the small intestine. J Clin Invest 1977;59:1158–1166.

60 Ojetti V, Pitocco D, Scarpellini E, Zaccardi F, et al: Small bowel bacterial overgrowth and type 1 diabetes. Eur Rev Med Pharmacol Sci 2009;13:419–423.

61 Resmini E, Parodi A, Savarino V, Greco A, et al: Evidence of prolonged oro-cecal transit time and small intestinal bacterial overgrowth in acromegalic patients. J Clin Endocrinol Metab 2007;92:2119–2124.

62 Strid H, Simren M, Stotzer PO, Ringstrom G, et al: Patients with chronic renal failure have abnormal small intestinal motility and a high prevalence of small intestinal bacterial overgrowth. Digestion 2003;67:129–137.

63 George NS, Sankineni A, Parkman HP: Small intestinal bacterial overgrowth in gastroparesis. Dig Dis Sci 2012, E-pub ahead of print.

64 Tarnopolsky MA, Pearce E, Matteliano A, James C, et al: Bacterial overgrowth syndrome in myotonic muscular dystrophy is potentially treatable. Muscle Nerve 2010;42:853–855.

65 Reddymasu SC, McCallum RW: Small intestinal bacterial overgrowth in gastroparesis: are there any predictors? J Clin Gastroenterol 2010;44:e8–e13.

66 Layritano EC, Bilotti AL, Gabrielli M, Scarpellini E, et al: Association between hypothyroidism and small intestinal bacterial overgrowth. J Clin Endocrinol Metab 2007;92:4180–4184.

67 Marie I, Ducrotté P, Denis P, Menard JF, et al: Small intestinal bacterial overgrowth in systemic sclerosis. Rheumatology 2009;48:1314–1319.

68 Parodi A, Sessarego M, Greco A, Bazzica M, et al: Small intestinal bacterial overgrowth in patients suffering from scleroderma: clinical effectiveness of its eradication. Am J Gastroenterol 2008;103:1257–1262.

69 Krishnamurthy S, Kelly MM, Rohrmann CA, Schuffler MD: Jejunal diverticulosis: a heterogeneous disorder caused by a variety of abnormalities of smooth muscle or myenteric plexus. Gastroenterology 1983;85:538–547.

Eamonn M.M. Quigley, MD, FRCP, FACP, FACG, FRCPI
Division of Gastroenterology, The Methodist Hospital
6550 Fannin St., SM 2001
Houston, TX 77030 (USA)
E-Mail equigley@tmhs.org

Quigley EMM, Hongo M, Fukudo S (eds): Functional and GI Motility Disorders.
Front Gastrointest Res. Basel, Karger, 2014, vol 33, pp 65–81 (DOI: 10.1159/000356745)

When and How Should We Study Colonic Motility?

Shin Fukudo · Takatsugu Machida · Yuka Endo · Tomotaka Shoji · Michiko Kano · Motoyori Kanazawa

Department of Behavioral Medicine, Tohoku University Graduate School of Medicine, and Department of Psychosomatic Medicine, Tohoku University Hospital, Sendai, Japan

Abstract

The colon has an autonomic activity owing to the concerted actions of the interstitial cells of Cajal, the enteric nervous system (especially myentric plexus and submucosal plexus), and smooth muscle cells. Changes in colonic motility are perceived centrally and can affect the neurons in the central nervous system. Conversely, the central nervous system can affect colonic motility via hormonal and neural signals. These reciprocal relations between the brain and the colon are known as the brain-gut interactions. Normal colonic motility consists of segmental contractions, propulsion, and high-amplitude propagating contractions. Physical stimulation of the internal lumen of the colon causes a reflex action and gastrointestinal perception. This activity comprises the peristaltic reflex, colo-colonic inhibitory reflex, and colonic perception. Several methods have been developed for observing colonic motility in the human body. Barostat and gastrointestinal manometry are suitable for the analysis of the gastrointestinal wall motion, while the analysis of gastrointestinal transit can be performed using radioisotopes, radiopaque markers, and the hydrogen breath test. There are various diseases based on the pathology and/or pathophysiology of colonic motility. They are chronic intestinal pseudo-obstruction, megacolon, colonic inertia, Hirschsprung's disease, colonic diverticula, colonic motility disorders due to systemic diseases, functional constipation, functional diarrhea, and irritable bowel syndrome. Thus, the physiology of colonic motility and pathology are gradually being elucidated. Functional investigations of motility in order to clarify pathological colonic motility are progressing. The ultimate goal is a treatment that is highly rational and highly effective in colonic motility disorders. It is important to identify the key molecules and disordered levels in the brain, autonomic nervous system, or enteric nervous system. A new technique is therefore required to address the whole understanding of disorders of colonic motility.

The colon has an autonomic activity due to the concerted actions of the interstitial cells of Cajal, the enteric nervous system (especially the myentric plexus and submucosal plexus), and smooth muscle cells [1]. Changes in colonic motility are perceived centrally and can affect the neurons in the central nervous system. Conversely, the central nervous system can affect colonic motility via hormonal and neural signals. These reciprocal relations between the brain and the colon are known as the brain-gut interactions. The neural pathways that connect the central nervous system to the colon comprise the extrinsic neurons of the gastrointestinal system. Extrinsic nerve fibers are known as autonomic nervous system [2]. They are classified into sympathetic division and parasympathetic divisions, and both of them contain efferent fibers and afferent fibers. When discussing autonomic regulation of the colon, the broadest definition includes all of the afferent and efferent signals from the central neurons, extrinsic neurons, and enteric nervous system. The strictest definition includes only the efferent signals from the extrinsic neurons. Functions that are unique to the enteric nervous system and especially to the myenteric plexus are also frequently referred to as gastrointestinal autonomic functions. In this chapter, we discuss colonic motility based on the broadest definition of autonomic regulation from the perspective of a biological system.

The Physiology of Colonic Motility

Specific Structure of the Colon

Gastrointestinal motility is caused by the contraction and relaxation of the inner circular muscle and the outer longitudinal muscle of the intestinal wall [1]. The structure of the muscular layer, however, differs markedly between the small intestine and the colon. The external longitudinal muscle does not cover the whole circumference of the colon, and taenia coli are formed through the aggregation of the longitudinal muscle in 3 places, namely in the area attached to the peritoneum, the area attached to the omentum, and at a location in between. Clinically, when the transverse colon is reached during colonoscopy, the shape of the lumen is easily recognized as approximating a triangle, and the external longitudinal muscle exists at all points of the triangle.

Electrophysiology of the Colon

Due to ion gradients, the interior of the smooth muscle cell membrane is negatively charged, and depolarization occurs repeatedly at a characteristic rhythm at 3- to 10-second intervals in all regions of the gastrointestinal system. This is known as electrical control activity (ECA) [3]. This change in the potential can also be measured extracellularly, and in the duodenum it happens 12 times a minute. ECA alone does not produce contractions; the electrical response activity (ERA) that is superimposed on the ECA causes the initiation of smooth muscle contractions. In the colon, ERAs (spike activity) that are superimposed on individual ECAs are known as short spike bursts and cause rhythmic segmentation. In contrast, spikes that are continuously superimposed on several ECAs and are generated repeatedly every 4 to 15 min are known as long spike bursts, which participate in propulsion. Migrating spike bursts are not related to ECA and occur when a high-frequency spike propagates in the rostral to caudal direction, and these spikes participate in mass movement [1]. The interstitial cells of Cajal generate pacemaker potentials by regularly undergoing repeated depolarization, thereby creating the source of small intestinal and colonic motility.

Molecular Mechanism of the Smooth Muscle Contraction

The molecular mechanism of smooth muscle motility has been clarified in greater detail [4]. Acetylcholine, the major excitatory neurotransmitter, binds to muscarinic M3 receptors and activates phospholipase C via coupled Go-proteins to create diacylglycerol and inositol trisphosphate (IP3). IP3 binds to the smooth muscle cell sarcoplasmic reticulum and releases stored calcium (Ca^{2+}) into the cytoplasm. Ca^{2+} binds to calmodulin, which, in turn, binds to myosin light chain kinase and activates it, which causes structural changes in myosin. Myosin then binds to actin and the smooth muscle cell contracts. In contrast, noradrenaline increases cytoplasmic cyclic adenosine monophosphate (cAMP) via β_2-receptors, Gs proteins, and adenylate cyclase. Cytoplasmic cAMP then activates cAMP-dependent protein kinase, which phosphorylates myosin light chain kinase, decreasing its ability to bind to calmodulin, and the result is the relaxation of smooth muscle cells. Nitric oxide formed from arginine by nitric oxide synthase also increases cyclic guanosine monophosphate (cGMP) through cytoplasmic guanylate cyclase, which activates cGMP-dependent protein kinase, which in turn causes a decrease in the intracellular Ca^{2+} concentration, resulting in the relaxation of smooth muscle cells. Several existing endogenous and exogenous substances influence smooth muscle motility, and the direction of action (i.e. contraction or relaxation) is determined by what changes are ultimately induced by the molecules inside the smooth muscle cells.

Patterns of Small Intestinal Motility in Comparison to Colonic Motility

In comparison to colonic motility, the character of normal small intestinal motility is described as follows. Normal small intestinal motility [3, 5, 6] shows completely different patterns in the fasted and postprandial states. In the fasted state, a period of absent contractions (phase I) is followed by a period of unsynchronized contractions (phase II) and a subsequent burst of regular, strong contractions at a frequency of 11–12 cycles a minute (phase III), during which the contents are propelled caudally. These migrating (interdigestive) motor complexes are repeated every 90–160 min. In the postprandial state, continuous irregular movements that resemble phase II contractions (fed pattern) occur for 2–3 h. The fed pattern terminates with complete emptying of the gastric contents and phase III-like contractions of the small intestine, followed by a transition to fasting state motility.

Patterns of Colonic Motility

Normal colonic motility [7–10] consists of 3 components. The first is rhythmic segmentation that creates the saccular-shaped colonic haustra, and this is the most common. Based on the intraluminal pressure, pressure waves from sequentially arranged intraluminal pressure sensors enable the formation of either mutually independent movements or simultaneously increased pressure. The second component is propulsion, in which the pressure waves move sequentially along the intraluminal pressure sensors on the long axis of the colon. While antegrade peristalsis can frequently be seen in the descending colon, retrograde peristalsis is frequently observed in the ascending colon. The third component is mass movement that is thought to contribute to defecation and only occurs a few times a day. These movements are known as high-amplitude propagating contractions, and they consist of high-pressure propulsive movements directed caudally (fig. 1) [11].

Neural Control of Colonic Motility

The most important structure that controls these gastrointestinal movements is the myenteric plexus, which lies between the external longitudinal muscle and the internal circular muscle [1]. The myenteric plexus contains an abundance of neurotransmitters such as acetylcholine, noradrenaline, serotonin (5-hydroxytryptamine, 5-HT), vasoactive intestinal peptide, nitric oxide, and cholecystokinin. These neurotransmitters bring about various changes in the smooth muscle cell membrane potential, which regulates autonomic gastrointestinal motility. The neurons in the myenteric plexus receive projections from the extrinsic neurons whose signals originate from the central nervous system [1]. The fibers of the extrinsic neurons are either sympathetic or parasympathetic. Sympathetic nerves have postganglionic fibers that release noradrenaline, which suppresses colonic motility. Meanwhile, the preganglionic fibers of the parasympathetic nerves release acetylcholine, which promotes colonic motility.

Sensorimotor Coordination of the Colon

Physical stimulation of the internal lumen of the colon causes a reflex action and gastrointestinal perception [12]. This activity comprises (1) the peristaltic reflex, (2) the colo-colonic inhibitory reflex, and (3) colonic perception.

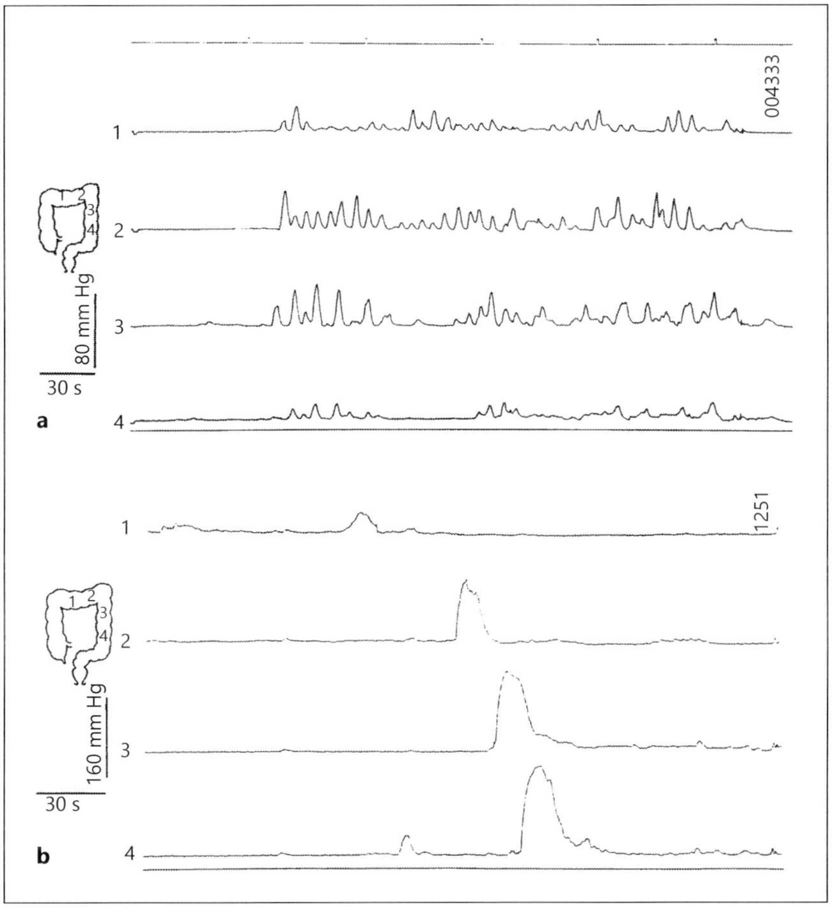

Fig. 1. Colonic intraluminal pressure in a healthy individual. **a** Segmental contractions of the colon. **b** High-amplitude propagating contractions. From Narducci et al. [11], with permission.

The Peristaltic Reflex

First, the peristaltic reflex is generated as follows: stimulation of the colonic mucosa by the influx of feces or gas stimulates enterochromaffin cells and releases 5-HT in the mucosa of the colon. Released 5-HT stimulates the intrinsic primary afferent neurons which have bipolar axons in the myenteric plexus with oral and aboral projections. On the oral side, the 5-HT interneuron is stimulated, and 5-HT is released to the synapse with the AH type 2 neuron. This is the colonic motor neuron and 5-HT3 and 5-HT4 receptors on the cell membrane play an important role in mediating acetylcholine release [13]. Thus, the neurotransmitter acetylcholine is released and causes ascending circular muscle contractions. On the other hand at the aboral side, the inhibitory neuron such as a nitric oxide neuron is stimulated, and descending circular muscle relaxation occurs. This peristaltic reflex makes the bowel contents migrate in the rostral to caudal direction [1].

The Colo-Colonic Inhibitory Reflex

Next, the colo-colonic inhibitory reflex occurs when the bowel receives distension stimuli from the influx of feces and gas. Then, the parallel receptor of the sensory nerve endings, which have their cell bodies in the myenteric plexus, are stimulated, and a signal is transmitted via the nicotinic receptor due to acetylcholine release at the sympathetic ganglia in the celiac ganglion, the superior mesenteric ganglia, or the inferior mesenteric ganglia [13]. When the inhibitory neurotransmitter noradrenaline, which suppresses acetylcholinergic neurons, is released at these sympathetic postganglionic neurons, it causes colonic relaxation [13]. Somatostatin and neuropeptide Y are also known to be present in postganglionic neurons. The parallel receptor in the intrinsic sensory neurons does not fire in response to active contraction of the circular muscle and is responsible for monitoring the state of bowel relaxation and contraction [13].

Colonic Perception

When distension stimuli increase, colonic perception is ultimately produced [12]. The spinal sensory neurons, which have receptors arranged serially in the longitudinal muscle, fire and transmit a signal via the viscerosomatic neurons that lie between the dorsal spinal nerve root and the posterior horn of the spinal cord [12]. Their axons ascend via the contralateral spinothalamic tract and spinoreticular tract and cause central visceral sensations (fig. 2) [14]. In other words, luminal stimuli send signals which enable monitoring of visceral events, in addition to reflex actions, to the central nervous system; in this manner, either a high-intensity stimulus or a low sensory threshold will give rise to colonic perception [12].

Measuring Colonic Motility in Humans

Several methods have been developed for observing colonic motility in the human body. The barostat [15–17] and gastrointestinal manometry [5–11] are suitable for the analysis of the gastrointestinal wall motion, while the analysis of gastrointestinal transit can be performed using radioisotopes [3, 18], radiopaque markers [19], and the hydrogen breath test [20]. Electromyograms [21] were used to analyze the source of colonic motility, which is rarely measured in humans.

Barostat

The barostat has a soft plastic bag that is inserted into the colon to perform detailed analysis of colonic motility, and the bag volume, pressure, and compliance are mea-

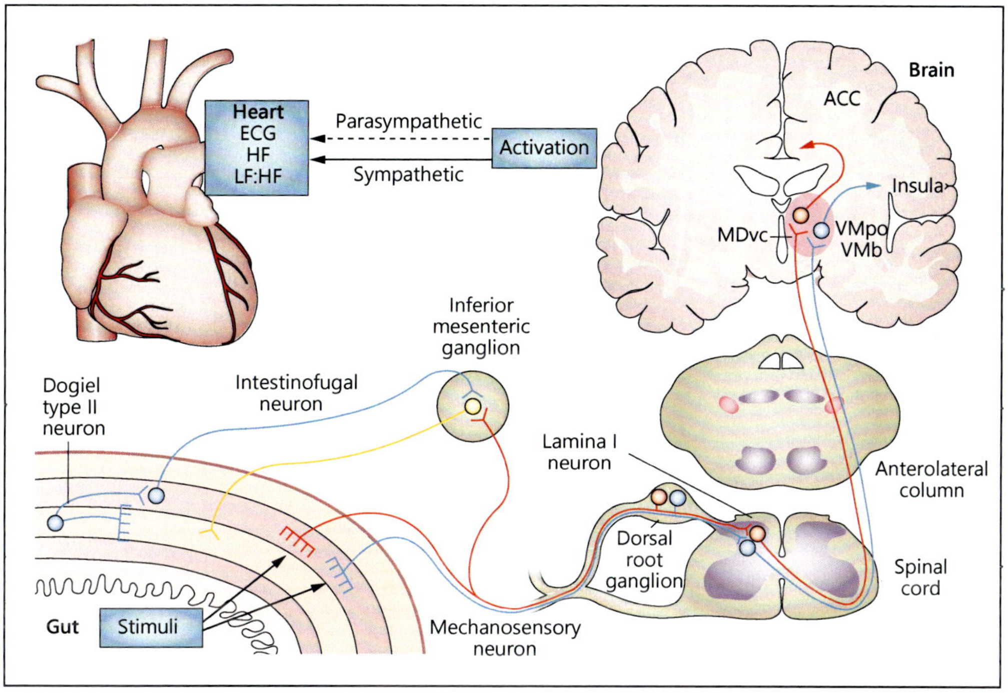

Fig. 2. Colonic perception pathway and autonomic efferent activation. The nociceptive signals from the colorectum ascend the fine sympathetic afferent fibers that pass the dorsal root ganglia. These primary afferent neurons have synapses with the second-order neurons in the lamina I of the dorsal horn of the spinal cord. The visceral afferent signals via lamina I pass the ventrocaudal part of medial dorsal nucleus (MDvc) and the ventral medial nucleus/posterior part of ventromedial nucleus (VMpo-VMb) of the thalamus. Pathways bypassing the thalamus via parabrachial nucleus, hypothalamus and amygdala are also present. The signals are processed in the homeostatic afferent network and emotional afferent network including insula and anterior cingulate cortex (ACC). Then, autonomic efferent pathways are activated and result in cardiac sympathetic arousal detected by an increase in the low frequency:high frequency (LF:HF) ratio and/or cardiac vagal withdrawal detected by a decrease in the HF component of heart rate variability. From Fukudo [14], with permission.

sured under computer control [9, 15]. Although it is possible to use a barostat in the small intestine, its use is limited to research. One advantage of the barostat is that, not only can it detect contractions that occlude the lumen, but it can also detect contractions that do not occlude the lumen, changes in colonic wall tension, and particularly relaxation responses. A further advantage of the barostat includes its ability to quantitatively assess visceral perception [15]. Excluding the three colonic movements mentioned here, other aspects of gastrointestinal motility can be measured simultaneously. However, such measurement is difficult, and it is impossible to accurately measure the pressure of contractions that occlude the lumen.

Measuring colonic wall tension requires application of static low pressure to the colon [15]. There are two methods for supplying static low pressure. One method involves applying a static pressure of 10–12 mm Hg to a bag, and the other involves applying a static pressure equal to minimal distending pressure (MDP) + 2 mm Hg. Normally, pressure is increased from 0 in 1–2 mm Hg increments, and MDP is defined as the lowest pressure at which respiratory movement can be detected on the colon capacity curve. For this reason, when using the method that applies a fixed pressure of MDP + 2 mm Hg, the pressure differs between subjects.

Colonic capacity is reduced if the colonic wall is tense, and it increases when the colonic wall is relaxed [15]. Normally, basic measurements are performed for more than 15 min, a stimulus is applied, and changes in colonic capacity are observed. In addition, it is possible to analyze long-term changes in colonic wall tension as well as brief contractions. Waves with a brief capacity change of more than 10% should be extracted from the long-term colonic capacity curve as phasic volume events.

Two methods are available for assessing colonic perception: pressure loading and volume loading [15]. Pressure loading is a means of detecting whether subjects are aware of visceral perception when the internal pressure of the bag is increased by a certain degree. Similarly, volume loading is an approach for detecting whether subjects are aware of visceral perception when the internal volume of the bag is increased by a certain degree. Pressure loading is considered a more objective measure than volume loading because a variation exists between subjects in terms of the capacity of the human colon. To measure perception using pressure loading, the bag is inflated at the maximum rate of approximately 40 ml/s. Thus, it is not possible to perform accurate measurements when the bag is inflated slowly. A few stimulation methods are available for measuring perception. The duration of the first stimulus is 30–60 s, and a stimulus interval of 30–60 s is preferred. Following a gradual increase in the pressure stimulus, it is recommended that stimulation that accurately determines the pain threshold should fluctuate at a pressure close to the pain threshold [15].

Colonic Manometry

Colonic manometry [7–11] is used to analyze the pattern of wall motion. It is accomplished by continuously measuring intraluminal pressure for prolonged periods of observation using a pressure transducer at the sphincter or under conditions such as rhythmic segmentation that roughly resembles a closed-loop obstruction. This enables detailed analysis of colonic wall motion. Methods of accomplishing sensor placement to achieve colonic intraluminal pressure measurements [7–11] include colonoscopy, use of guidewires, and insertion into the colon through a sliding tube. The region most frequently measured is the sigmoid colon, but it is also possible to measure the intraluminal pressure of the descending colon, the transverse colon, and the ascending colon. The advantage of colonic intraluminal pressure measurement is that it is useful for detecting contraction of the colonic wall at different sites. Its disadvantage, however, is that it cannot be used to detect contractions that do not occlude the lumen, changes in colonic wall tension, and particularly relaxation responses.

Radioisotope Method

Substances that have been labeled using radionuclides are administered to the colon, and their migration is imaged by a gamma camera [3]. This is the method for analyzing migration dynamics. The investigation is conducted by orally administering a capsule which releases substance labeled with radiotracer in the terminal ileum [18].

Radiopaque Markers

Radiopaque markers are administered orally, and plain abdominal radiography obtained at fixed intervals enable observation of gastrointestinal transit [19]. It is also possible to observe transit through each constituent part of the intestine, but radiopaque markers are most suitable for diagnosing the presence of delayed transit throughout the entire gastrointestinal tract or colon.

Hydrogen Breath Test

When nonabsorbable carbohydrates reach the colon, they are metabolized by anaerobic bacteria, and hydrogen gas is produced. Based on this principle, nonabsorbable carbohydrates such as lactulose are administered and orally exhaled hydrogen gas concentration measured over time. The time from administration until a marked increase in hydrogen gas concentration occurs is considered the orocecal transit time [20]. The orocecal transit time also includes the small intestinal transit time, and it is also influenced by gastric emptying time. In addition, if the anaerobic bacteria from the colon invade the small intestine and bacterial overgrowth occurs, the hydrogen breath test will not accurately reflect the orocecal transit time. The hydrogen breath test provides collateral evidence for the time it takes for the leading portion of the food bolus to reach the cecum. However, it is not possible to use this test to determine whether or not the main portion of the food bolus or the whole food bolus has migrated into the colon.

Pathology of Colonic Motility

Chronic Intestinal Pseudo-Obstruction

Chronic intestinal pseudo-obstruction is the most serious small intestinal and colonic motility disorder [22, 23]. This disease is classified into visceral neuropathy or visceral myopathy depending on whether the dysfunction involves mainly neurons or

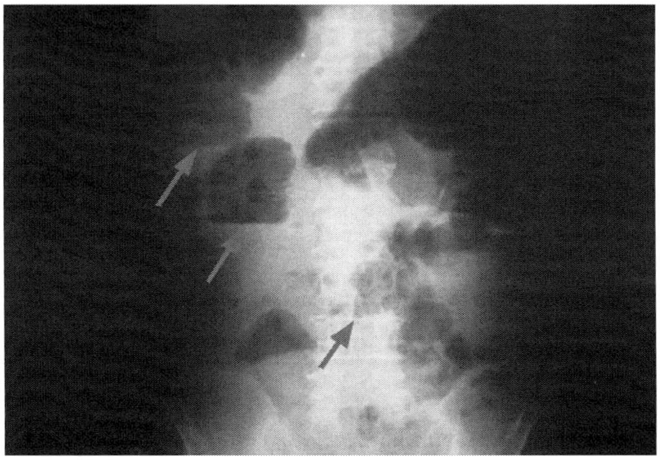

Fig. 3. Plain abdominal radiography of a patient with chronic idiopathic intestinal pseudo-obstruction. Obvious bowel dilation and the formation of air-fluid levels (arrows) were seen.

muscle. Individuals with detectable primary diseases including systemic sclerosis, amyloidosis, and neurodegenerative disorders are simply referred to as having chronic intestinal pseudo-obstruction. Conversely, when the primary disease cannot be identified, the idiopathic variant is known as chronic idiopathic intestinal pseudo-obstruction [23]. In some cases, lesions are located mainly in the small intestine, while in other cases, they are mainly in the colon. With disease progression or more extensive disease, maximum depression of intestinal wall motion results and patients present with megaduodenum or megacolon. Other than constipation, symptoms include abdominal distension, pain, nausea, and vomiting. In addition, bacterial overgrowth occurs due to the stasis of the intestinal contents, and patients commonly present with diarrhea due to the production of bacterial toxins such as organic acids and *Clostridium difficile* toxin. Gas accumulation and air-fluid levels can be observed in the small and large bowel on plain abdominal radiographs (fig. 3), in the dilated small and large bowel on computed tomography. In terms of the small intestinal intraluminal pressure, the frequency of the phase III activity is reduced. In some cases, nonpropagating burst activities with amplitudes above 20 mm Hg and with contraction frequency of 10–12 cpm are sustained for at least 2 min. Reduced motility or no transition from the fasting pattern to fed pattern are noted during the period in which movements generally occurred. If the condition worsens, contractions will largely disappear and the small intestine and colon will dilate.

Megacolon

Intestinal hypomotility is accompanied by dilation of the colon and rectum. Pathological investigations conducted to date have shown degeneration of the noncholinergic, nonadrenergic inhibitory neurons in the myenteric plexus.

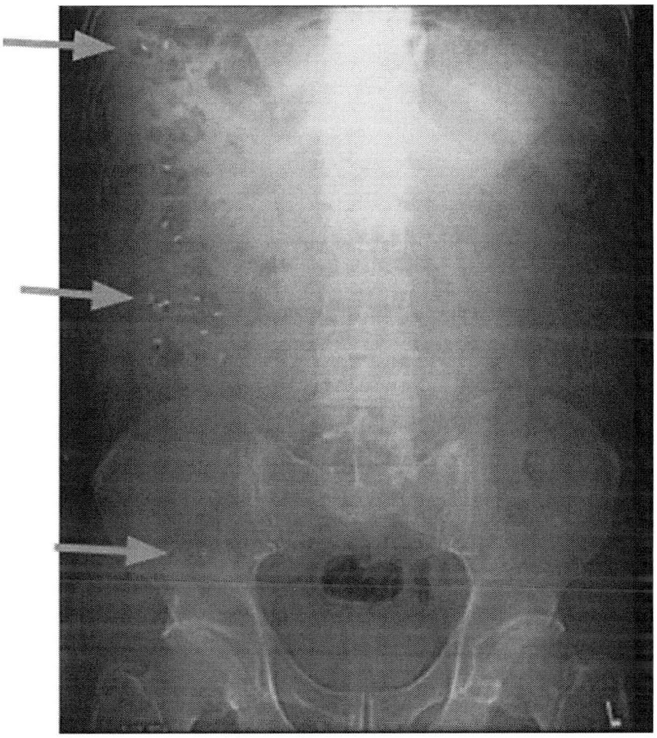

Fig. 4. Plain abdominal radiography of a patient with colonic inertia in the standing position. On day 9 of radiopaque marker administration, the markers (arrows) remained in the ascending colon. In normal individuals, up to 100% of radiopaque markers are excreted by day 7.

Colonic Inertia

This disorder represents a more severe form of functional constipation and is common in young women, whereas colonic hypomotility is not usually accompanied by marked dilation of the colon [24] (fig. 4). Colonic inertia is also known as severe idiopathic constipation [25, 26]. Gastrointestinal transit time is normal up to the cecum when measured using radiopaque markers. In contrast, the time required for colonic emptying is markedly delayed. Small intestinal manometry shows a normal pattern, but in terms of colonic intraluminal pressure, there is a reduced incidence of rhythmic segmentation, which is not induced by the administration of cholinergic agents. Pathological investigations conducted to date show degeneration of the cholinergic excitatory neurons in the myenteric plexus [25].

Hirschsprung's Disease

Hirschsprung's disease involves denervation and narrowing of the distal rectum continuing to the anus due to a lack of ganglion cells in the submucosal plexus and the myenteric plexus in the lower gastrointestinal tract. Patients present with congenital megacolon and dilation of the proximal digestive tract [3]. Hirschsprung's disease is frequently complicated by multiple endocrine neoplasia type 2, which is hereditary, and also by Waardenburg syndrome, which presents with deafness and dyschromatosis. According to genetic linkage studies, abnormalities of the ret, endothelin B receptor, and endothelin 3 genes have been detected, and these genes have been identified as participating in the rostral to caudal formation of the neural crest.

Outlet Obstruction

In this condition, normal evacuation is not possible due to functional or organic disorders of the anorectum and/or pelvic floor, and constipation occurs as a result. Measurements of gastrointestinal transit times are normal up to the rectum when measured using radiopaque markers, but the time required for rectal emptying is markedly delayed. Abnormalities of the rectoanal reflex or the inability of the striated muscle of the external anal sphincter to relax are observed on anorectal manometry. Although outlet obstruction is not a typical colonic motility disorder, it frequently presents a problem in the differential diagnosis of constipation.

Colonic Diverticula

Colonic diverticula are thought to form when the mucosa prolapses through the bowel wall in the weak area where the mesenteric artery penetrates the muscularis propria. This occurs in the direction of the peritoneal cavity due to increased colonic intraluminal pressure. Normally, the frequency of pressure waves of greater than 20 mm Hg is increased 2- to 3-fold.

Colonic Motility Disorders due to Systemic Diseases

Sometimes, stool abnormalities such as diarrhea and constipation or an alternating diarrhea and constipation occur in a variety of systemic diseases. The causes are divided into those believed to be directly related to the pathophysiology of the underlying disease and those believed to be indirectly related.

A typical example of a directly related cause is constipation in Parkinson's disease. An investigation of patients with Parkinson's disease who presented with constipation revealed a deficiency of dopaminergic neurons in the myenteric plexus in 82% of patients [27], compared with the healthy regions of the colon in patients with idiopathic severe constipation or those with colonic cancer. In Parkinson's disease, the dopamine concentration in the muscularis layer is also reduced, and Lewy bodies, which are not observed in the normal myenteric plexus, are frequently observed. The brains of Parkinson's disease patients are deficient in dopaminergic neurons in the substantia nigra. Lewy bodies, which are homogenous intracellular inclusion bodies, are characteristic pathological findings. In Parkinson's disease, therefore, pathological findings exist in both the nerves of the brain and those of the gastrointestinal system.

In terms of direct relationships, there are cases of diarrhea in diabetic patients with autonomic neuropathy, and there are also cases of lower gastrointestinal tract motility disorders as a side effect of medication. Antipsychotic drugs (e.g. chlorpromazine or haloperidol), antidepressants (e.g. imipramine or amitriptyline), and antiparkinsonian agents (e.g. trihexyphenidyl or biperiden) have anticholinergic effects and can cause constipation as a side effect. Levodopa is a dopaminergic agent and thus shows inhibitory effects on colonic motility, and it can also cause constipation as a side effect. When the suppression of colonic motility as a side effect of medication is considered together with the pathophysiology related directly to the systemic disease, it is easy to see that constipation is further exacerbated.

Functional Constipation

The definition of constipation is complex but it is accurately defined in the Rome III criteria, which constitute the international diagnostic standards for functional gastrointestinal disorders [28, 29]. In the Rome III criteria, functional constipation is defined as follows:

1 Must include two or more of the following:
   a Straining during at least 25% of defecations
   b Lumpy or hard stools in at least 25% of defecations
   c Sensation of incomplete evacuation for at least 25% of defecations
   d Sensation of anorectal obstruction/blockage for at least 25% of defecations
   e Manual maneuvers to facilitate at least 25% of defecations (e.g. digital evacuation, support of the pelvic floor)
   f Fewer than three defecations per week
2 Loose stools are rarely present without the use of laxatives
3 Insufficient criteria for irritable bowel syndrome

Criteria should be fulfilled for the last 3 months with symptom onset at least 6 months prior to diagnosis.

Typically, radiopaque markers disclose slow transit of the colon in patients with functional constipation [29].

Irritable Bowel Syndrome

In the Rome III diagnostic criteria [28, 29], IBS is defined by recurrent abdominal pain or discomfort at least 3 days per month in the last 3 months associated with 2 or more of the following: improvement with defecation, onset associated with a change in fre-

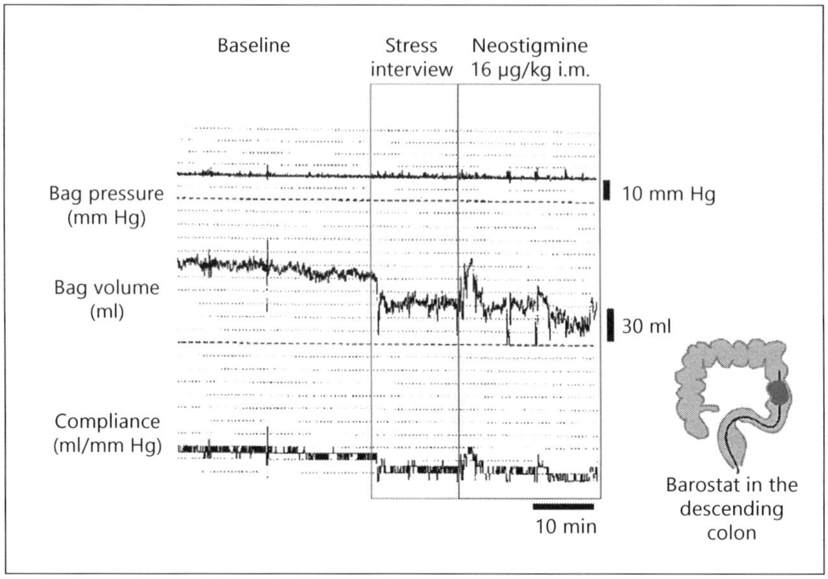

Fig. 5. Stress-induced contraction of the colon in a 30-year-old male patient with IBS. A barostat bag was placed in the descending colon of a patient with IBS with diarrhea. The bag pressure was kept at 10 mm Hg by barostat equipment. Note that the bag volume showed approximately 60 ml at baseline and around 30 ml at stress interview. Intramuscular injection of acetylcholinesterase inhibitor induced initial increase in bag volume followed by some lumen-occlusive contractions of the colon. From Fukudo [17], with permission.

quency of stool, and/or onset associated with a change in form (appearance) of stool. Criteria should be fulfilled for the last 3 months with symptom onset at least 6 months prior to diagnosis. Typical patients with IBS show exaggerated colonic motor response to various physiological stimuli including psychological stress (fig. 5) [7, 10], distention of the colorectum [30, 31], meals [31], a cholinesterase inhibitor [10] and corticotropin-releasing hormone (fig. 6) [32]. Dysmotility of the small bowel such as clustered contractions has also (but not always) been reported [5, 6]. Key pathophysiological factors in IBS also include visceral hypersensitivity, including a decreased perception threshold and an exaggerated subjective feeling of visceral perception [33]. IBS is characterized by dysfunctional autonomic regulation and brain-gut interactions [14]. Allostatic load of the regional brain, autonomic nervous system, and/or myenteric plexus are/is suggested to be the responsible pathophysiology of IBS [14].

Conclusion

The physiology of colonic motility and pathology are gradually being elucidated. Functional investigations of motility in order to clarify pathological colonic motility are progressing. The ultimate goal is treatment that is highly rational and highly ef-

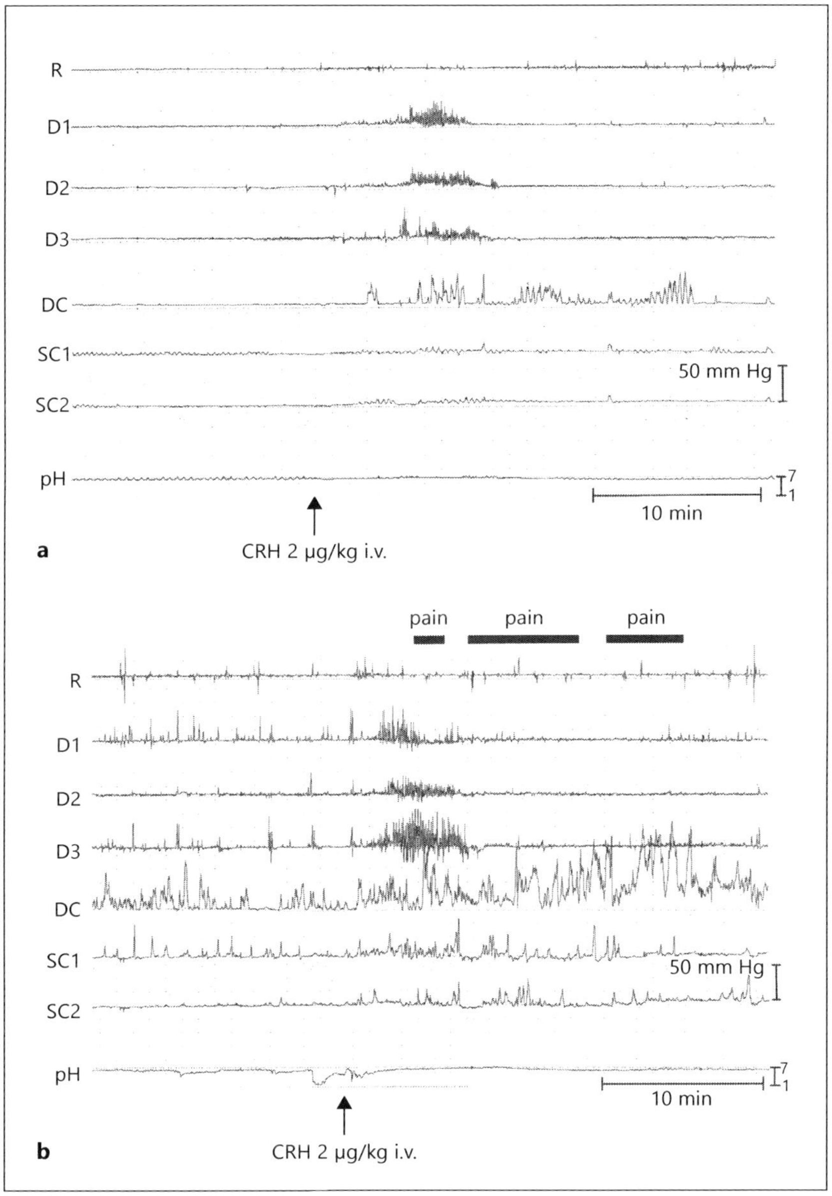

Fig. 6. CRH-induced contraction of the colon. **a** Colonic contractions and duodenal phase III were evoked in healthy normal men. **b** Administration of CRH stimulated the colon, particularly the descending colon, and evoked duodenal phase III in patients with IBS. This patient complained of abdominal pain during the periods expressed by solid bars. R = Respiration; D1 = duodenal bulb/antrum (60 cm); D2 = proximal second portion of the duodenum (65 cm); D3 = distal second portion of the duodenum (70 cm); DC = descending colon (60 cm); SC1 = proximal sigmoid colon (55 cm); SC2 = mid-sigmoid colon (50 cm); pH = duodenal pH (75 cm). Numbers in parentheses indicates rough distance from the mouth or anus. Arrow indicates intravenous administration of 2 µg/kg of human CRH. From Fukudo [17], with permission.

fective in colonic motility disorders. It is important to identify the key molecules and disordered levels in the brain, autonomic nervous system, or enteric nervous system. A new technique is therefore required to address this issue.

Acknowledgements

This research was supported by Grant-in-Aid for Scientific Research from the Ministry of Education, Science, and Culture of Japan, and Grant-in-Aid for Scientific Research from the Ministry of Health, Welfare, and Labor of Japan.

References

1 Davison JS: Innervation of the gastrointestinal tract; in Christensen J, Wingate DL (eds): A Guide to Gastrointestinal Motility. Bristol, Wright, 1983, pp 1–47.

2 Horn JP, Swanson LW: The autonomic nervous system and the hypothalamus; in Kandel ER, Schwartz JH, Jessel TM, Spiegelbaum SA, Hudspeth AJ (eds): Principles of Neural Science, ed 5. New York, McGraw-Hill, 2013, pp 1056–1078.

3 Kumar D, Wingate D: An Illustrated Guide to Gastrointestinal Motility, ed 2. London, Churchil Livingstone, 1993.

4 Somlyo AP, Somlyo AV: Signal transduction and regulation in smooth muscle. Nature 1994;372:231–236.

5 Kellow JE, Phillips SF: Altered small bowel motility in irritable bowel syndrome is correlated with symptoms. Gastroenterology 1987;92:1885–1893.

6 Kellow JE, Gill RC, Wingate DL: Prolonged ambulant recordings of small bowel motility demonstrate abnormalities in the irritable bowel syndrome. Gastroenterology 1990;98:1208–1218.

7 Fukudo S, Suzuki J: Colonic motility, autonomic function, and gastrointestinal hormones under psychological stress on irritable bowel syndrome. Tohoku J Exp Med 1987;151:373–385.

8 Rogers J, Henry MM, Misiewicz JJ: Increased segmental activity and intraluminal pressures in the sigmoid colon of patients with the irritable bowel syndrome. Gut 1989;30:634–641.

9 Steadman CJ, Phillips SF, Camilleri M, Haddad AC, Hanson RB: Variation of muscle tone in the human colon. Gastroenterology 1991;101:373–381.

10 Fukudo S, Nomura T, Muranaka M, Taguchi F: Brain-gut response to stress and cholinergic stimulation in irritable bowel syndrome. J Clin Gastroenterol 1993;17:133–141.

11 Narducci F, Bassotti G, Gaburri M, Morelli A: Twenty four hour manometric recording of colonic motor activity in healthy man. Gut 1987;28:17–25.

12 Mayer EA, Raybould HE: Role of visceral afferent mechanisms in functional bowel disorders. Gastroenterology 1990;99:1688–1704.

13 Szurszewski JH, Miller SM: Physiology of prevertebral ganglia; in Johnson LR (ed): Physiology of the Gastrointestinal Tract, ed 3. New York, Raven, 1994, pp 795–877.

14 Fukudo S: IBS: Autonomic dysregulation in IBS. Nat Rev Gastroenterol Hepatol 2013;10:569–571.

15 Whitehead WE, Delvaux M: Standardization of barostat procedures for testing smooth muscle tone and sensory thresholds in the gastrointestinal tract. Dig Dis Sci 1997;42:223–241.

16 Sagami Y, Shimada Y, Tayama J, Nomura T, Satake M, Endo Y, Shoji T, Karahashi K, Hongo M, Fukudo S: Effect of a corticotropin releasing hormone receptor antagonist on colonic sensory and motor function in patients with irritable bowel syndrome. Gut 2004;53:958–964.

17 Fukudo S: Hypothalamic-pituitary-adrenal axis in gastrointestinal physiology; in Johnson L (ed): Physiology of the Gastrointestinal Tract, ed 5. Oxford, Elsevier, 2012, pp 795–815.

18 Cremonini F, Mullan BP, Camilleri M, Burton DD, Rank MR: Performance characteristics of scintigraphic transit measurements for studies of experimental therapies. Aliment Pharmacol Ther 2002;16: 1781–1790.

19 Hinton JM, Lennard-Jones JE, Young AC: A new method for studying gut transit times using radiopaque markers. Gut 1969;10:842–847.

20 Read NW: Measurement of small bowel transit in humans; in Kamm M, Lennard-Jones J (eds): Gastrointestinal Transit: Pathophysiology and Pharmacology. Petersfield, Wrightson Biomedical Publishing, 1991, pp 97–108.

21 Snape WJ Jr, Carlson GM, Cohen S: Colonic myoelectrical activity in the irritable bowel syndrome. Gastroenterology 1976;70:326–330.

22 Schuffler MD, Rohrmann CA, Chaffee RG, Brand DL, Delaney JH, Young JH: Chronic intestinal pseudo-obstruction. A report of 27 cases and review of the literature. Medicine 1981;60:173–196.
23 Stanghellini V, Camilleri M, Malagelada JR: Chronic idiopathic intestinal pseudo-obstruction: clinical and intestinal manometric findings. Gut 1987;28:5–12.
24 Watier A, Devroede G, Duranceau A, Abdel-Rahman M, Duguay C, Forand MD, Tétreault L, Arhan P, Lamarche J, Elhilali M: Constipation with colonic inertia: a manifestation of systemic disease? Dig Dis Sci 1983;28:1025–1033.
25 Krishnamurthy S, Schuffler MD, Rohrmann CA, Pope CE 2nd: Severe idiopathic constipation is associated with a distinctive abnormality of the colonic myenteric plexus. Gastroenterology 1985;88:26–34.
26 Wald A, Hinds JP, Caruana BJ: Psychological and physiological characteristics of patients with severe idiopathic constipation. Gastroenterology 1989;97:932–937.
27 Singaram C, Ashraf W, Gaumnitz EA, Torbey C, Sengupta A, Pfeiffer R, Quigley EM: Dopaminergic defect of enteric nervous system in Parkinson's disease patients with chronic constipation. Lancet 1995;346:861–864.
28 Drossman DA: The functional gastrointestinal disorders and the Rome III process. Gastroenterology 2006;130:1377–1390.
29 Longstreth GF, Thompson WG, Chey WD, Houghton LA, Mearin F, Spiller RC: Functional bowel disorders. Gastroenterology 2006;130:1480–1491.
30 Fukudo S, Kanazawa M, Kano M, Sagami Y, Endo Y, Utsumi A, Nomura T, Hongo M: Exaggerated motility of the descending colon with repetitive distention of the sigmoid colon in patients with irritable bowel syndrome. J Gastroenterol 2002;37(suppl 14):145–150.
31 Kanazawa M, Palsson OS, Thiwan SIM, Turner MJ, van Tilburg MAL, Gangarosa LM, Chitkara DK, Fukudo S, Drossman DA, Whitehead WE: Contributions of pain sensitivity and colonic motility to IBS symptom severity and predominant bowel habits. Am J Gastroenterol 2008;103:2550–2561.
32 Fukudo S, Nomura T, Hongo M: Impact of corticotropin-releasing hormone on gastrointestinal motility in normal subjects and patients with irritable bowel syndrome. Gut 1998;42:845–849.
33 Bouin M, Plourde V, Boivin M, Riberdy M, Lupien F, Laganiere M, Verrier P, Poitras P: Rectal distention testing in patients with irritable bowel syndrome: sensitivity, specificity, and predictive values of pain sensory thresholds. Gastroenterology 2002;122:1771–1777.

Dr. Shin Fukudo
Department of Behavioral Medicine, Tohoku University Graduate School of Medicine
2-1 Seiryo-machi
Aoba-ku, Sendai 980-8575 (Japan)
E-Mail sfukudo@med.tohoku.ac.jp

Quigley EMM, Hongo M, Fukudo S (eds): Functional and GI Motility Disorders.
Front Gastrointest Res. Basel, Karger, 2014, vol 33, pp 82–94 (DOI: 10.1159/000356750)

Difficult Defecation: What Really Helps to Assess Dysfunction and Guide Therapy

Enrico Stefano Corazziari

Dipartimento di Medicina Interna e Specialità Mediche, Università Sapienza ROMA, Roma, Italy

Abstract

Difficult or silent, unexpressed, and complicated defecation is assessed with a proper medical history, physical examination of the anorectum, as well as the evaluation of patient's behavior developed in response to, or as cause of, the disturbance. No particular investigations are required in the patient not presenting alarm symptoms or risk factors and the initial treatment based on bowel education, proper diet/fiber and laxatives is usually successfull. Patients who do not benefit from initial treatment undergo successive diagnostic steps aiming to identify the basic pathophysiological alterations, either related to colorectal transit or defecatoriy mechanism, amenable to treatment.

Clinical Presentation

Difficult defecation can be: (1) expressed by the patient as a feeling of incomplete evacuation; defecatory straining; frequent and repeated evacuations of small insufficient amounts of stools; a sensation of anorectal obstruction; hard, pellety or lumpy, stools (type 1–3 of the Bristol Stool Scale); the need for manual maneuvers to facilitate defecation (e.g. by applying pressure on the perineum anteriorly to the anus or through the posterior wall of the vagina or by digital evacuation); (2) silent, unexpressed, e.g. in children, subjects with cognitive defects or psychological disorders; habitual users of laxatives or enemas; (3) manifested by a complication, e.g. fecal incontinence or obstruction because of fecalomas in people affected by silent constipation.

Clinical Evaluation

Physician-Patient Relationship – A Biopsychosocial-Behavioral Approach to Patients

The first and fundamental step in the diagnostic approach is to obtain a proper medical history and perform a physical examination.

The diagnostic and therapeutic strategy should be based on a correct approach to the patient and a dialogue that will make it possible to identify, at the first encounter and when taking the history, all of the factors contributing to the disturbance, and not just the clinical history of the symptoms. It is important to evaluate the evolution of the disorder over time carefully in order to identify any behavioral habits developed by the patient either as a possible cause or a consequence of a usually long-standing condition.

Patient behavior is particularly important in the case of chronic constipation insofar as defecation involves the intervention of the voluntary sphere which, in its turn, is greatly conditioned by biological factors, the patient's psychological status and culture, and by his social and healthcare environment. For example, the pain caused by an anal fissure is a frequent biological reason for avoiding or postponing defecation; and the same may be true, for cultural reasons, if the toilet is not clean, for social or psychological reasons if it is not sufficiently private or acoustically insulated or for reasons of physical incapacity and/or cognitive impairment in bedridden, elderly subjects who are no longer independent. Behavior also interacts with the (self)-management and treatment of constipation, as in the case of a change in diet or, more frequently, false beliefs concerning the use of laxatives or enemas. One of the most deleterious preconceptions is that laxatives should be avoided altogether and replaced by an excessive use of dietary fibers and straining, or by the continuous use of herbs that frequently contain stimulating contact laxatives.

Physical Examination of the Perineum and the Anorectum

With the patient in the left lateral decubitus position and with the knees flexed on the chest, it is possible to observe the upward and downward movement of the perineum during simulated evacuation and maximal anal contraction. The perianal skin should be checked for fecal loss, and the anal reflex tested by gently pricking the perianal skin with a needle. During simulated evacuation, observe the degree of anal relaxation: if the anus remains open, it indicates neurogenic damage or the presence of anorectal mucosa prolapse. Digital examination is used to evaluate anal tone under basal conditions and during maximal contraction. Check whether the rectal ampulla is empty or contains feces. After an interval of 3 or more days since the last defecation, an empty ampulla indicates colonic slowing, and a full ampulla is suggestive of rectal slowing, and a massive fecal amount of fecaloma. The puborectalis muscle should be hooked by the intrarectal finger in order to verify whether inhibition occurs during simulated evacuation, and whether acute pain is felt when the muscle is palpated and compressed. The presence of rectoceles is evaluated with the finger turned anteriorly. A carefully performed digital examination is useful to detect dyssynergia with sensitivities and specificities of 75 and 87%, respectively [1].

A search should be made for associated anorectal conditions that can either alter, or are secondary to, the defecation act and may cause bowel and urinary disorders (table 1).

Table 1. Conditions associated with or complicating defecatory disorders

Related to defecatory straining
– Pathological hemorrhoids
– Anal fissure
– Rectal/anorectal intussusception; rectal prolapse
– Rectocele
– Solitary rectal ulcer
Related to fecal accumulation; fecalomas
– Distension and abdominal pain
– Intestinal occlusion/perforation
– Fecal incontinence
– Urinary retention

Rectoceles and Rectorectal Intussusception

Rectoceles and rectorectal intussusception are highly prevalent structural alterations, especially in women, but they are equally frequent in asymptomatic subjects and patients with chronic constipation [2, 3]. The natural history of chronic constipation (which often appears at a young age and lasts for decades) is indicative of the fact that disordered bowel movements with defecatory straining precede and favor the development of rectal disease which, in turn, can contribute to the worsening of defecatory difficulties, thus sustaining a vicious circle of constipation and alterations in rectal anatomy.

Pathological Hemorrhoids

Observational studies have not found that constipated patients are at any greater risk of developing pathological hemorrhoids [4] which, however, are often preceded by acute constipation and are probably caused by the effects of straining during defecation [5].

Anal Fissures

There is no greater risk of anal fissures associated with chronic constipation. The presence of a fissure favors the onset of acute constipation and, in some circumstances (for example, during infancy) can lead to chronic constipation.

Solitary Rectal Ulcer Syndrome

Solitary rectal ulcer syndrome is an infrequent condition characterized by inflammation and chronic ulceration of the rectum that is encountered in constipated patients who have difficulty in defecating. Its etiology is unknown, but it is found in the presence of constipation, increased pressure in the anal canal, and, in a large proportion of patients, rectorectal intussusception [6]. Therapy is aimed at treating constipation by reducing the consistency of hard feces and, in the presence of dyssynergic defecation, the restoration of abdominopelvic synergy [7].

Table 2. Alarm factors

An age of more than 50 years
Recent symptom onset
Rectal bleeding
Fever
Unintentional weight loss
Severe unstudied symptoms
Continuous symptoms
Symptoms causing awakenings
A family history of colorectal cancer, inflammatory bowel diseases, celiac disease, visceral neuromyopathies
Abnormal laboratory test values
Objective finding of an abdominal or rectal mass

Fecal Rectal Impaction and Incontinence

Fecal rectal impaction may prevent spontaneous defecation and lead to fecal incontinence, mainly in children and elderly subjects. However, fecal retention and the formation of fecalomas can occur at all ages (on average 60 years), and is more frequent in bedridden patients and those who use drugs that cause constipation [8]. In those who develop fecalomas located more proximally, perforation due to a stercoral ulcer is a rare and usually unforeseen event that accounts for 3% of all colonic perforation, usually in women with a long history of constipation.

In conclusion, the following are the main objectives a physician should bear in mind when first encountering the patient complaining of constipation: (1) establish a relationship of mutual trust; (2) determine the onset and evolution of the clinical condition; (3) find out why the patient decided to seek medical help for a condition that has lasted for so long; (4) evaluate all of the possible co-factors, i.e. the comorbidities and psychological, environmental, dietary and behavioral factors that, alone or in combination, commonly contribute to causing the overall clinical picture; (5) search for the presence of fecalomas or anorectal diseases; (6) ascertain whether the symptoms reported by the patient are compatible with the condition of chronic constipation [9] and require further diagnostic investigations.

Initial (Therapeutic) Approach to Patients with Difficult Defecation

In a minority of cases, the disorder may be secondary to clearly identifiable causal or predisposing factors, such as anatomical abnormalities, endocrine or metabolic diseases and constipating drug therapies; in the majority of cases, it is primary and functional.

Management cannot be generalized to all patients in a standard manner. It is usually recommended to adopt a diagnostic and therapeutic approach that can be based on a number of successive diagnostic steps and the sequential or combined use of different therapies. A careful clinical assessment of warning signs and symptoms or

Table 3. Clinically relevant conditions requiring focused diagnostic and therapeutic strategy

1	Presence of disturbances that significantly interfere with everyday activities
2	Persistence of disturbances due to an unsatisfactory or no response to dietary/behavioral therapy and laxatives
3	Onset or risk of complications such as fecal incontinence, anal fissures, hemorrhoids, a solitary rectal ulcer, or intestinal obstruction or perforation due to fecalomas
4	Need to avoid excessive straining when defecating, for example in the case of patients with cardiorespiratory insufficiency
5	Inability to manage bowel movements autonomously because of cognitive deficits or physical impairment

risk factors (alarm factors; table 2) is fundamental because, in their absence, no particular diagnostic investigation is required in patients aged less than 50 years except for a few laboratory tests (at the discretion of the physician) to evaluate hemoglobin, creatinine, blood glucose, thyroid function, serum levels of calcium and phosphate, and anti-transglutaminase antibodies. A detailed drug history should be obtained in order to identify the use of any drugs that can cause constipation and eliminate or replace them. Some constipating drugs cannot be discontinued, in which case it will be necessary to manage irreversible secondary constipation. A morphological study of the colon with barium contrast enema or colonoscopy is not required at this stage in patients aged <50 years and without any alarm factors.

The initial treatment of difficult defecation is based on a good physician-patient relationship and correct information being given to the patient. It is essential to explain the main functions of the colon and the recto-ano-pelvic apparatus, and the main mechanisms of continence and evacuation (and therefore the origin of any alterations), if possible by making use of simple anatomical drawings.

Most individuals with difficult defecation have mild and/or intermittent disorders and benefit from treatment based on the institution of a daily habit and bowel education, proper diet and fiber, and laxatives.

Further Diagnostic and Therapeutic Measures in Patients Who Do Not Benefit from Initial Treatment (Refractory Constipation)

In patients who do not benefit from initial treatment, the disturbance may be chronic and disabling, leading to a state of suffering or to conditions that predispose the patient to complications that require a more focused diagnostic and therapeutic strategy (table 3).

The main mechanisms that can lead to difficult defecation are slow colonic transit or altered recto-ano-pelvic function. Consequently, patients are classified into subtypes on the basis of their colorectal transit times and alterations in anorectal motor and sensory functions, bearing in mind that the different subtypes are not mutually exclusive but often overlapping.

The most widespread (but simplistic and often erroneous) interpretation is that the symptom complex of difficult defecation is due to anatomical or functional alterations in the anorectal-pelvic apparatus obstructing the passage of feces from the rectum to the anus. This has resulted in the use of the synonym 'obstructed defecation' but can actually be due to various alterations not caused by obstructive mechanisms, including fecal retention, megarectum, reduced evacuatory pressure, an alteration in the predefecatory colonic motor pattern, a reduction (or an increase) in the threshold of the defecatory stimulus, rectal hypersensitivity, or a central alteration in the perception of the defecatory stimulus. The presence of anatomical alterations such as rectoceles, rectoanal intussusception or pelvic dyssynergia per se does not explain the defecatory disturbances because the same alterations can also be found in asymptomatic subjects [2, 3].

The evidence that macrogol-based therapy resolves the defecatory symptoms among 75% of patients with rectoceles, rectorectal intussusception and functional recto-ano-pelvic dysfunctions by reducing fecal consistency [10] and improving colorectal transit demonstrates that while structural and functional alterations may contribute to defecatory dysfunction, they cannot be regarded as solely responsible in the majority of cases. Rather than being 'obstructed defecation', most of the instances would seem to be due to the fact that the patients' recto-ano-pelvic apparatus has difficulty in dealing with small, dehydrated nut-like feces.

It is important to emphasize that these two pathophysiologic mechanisms, slow transit and defecatory dysfunction, cannot be differentiated on the basis of symptoms or objective findings.

Slow colonic transit leads to dehydration, with the consequent formation of hard pellet-shaped feces that can only be expelled by means of considerable straining leading to incomplete rectal emptying; vice versa, ano-recto-pelvic alterations that do not allow satisfactory defecation or that induce patients to postpone defecating can cause slow colonic transit. The finding of feces in the ampulla upon rectal exploration is certainly a clue indicating rectal slowing, but does not indicate the presence or absence of colonic slowing. Finally, the same patient may be simultaneously affected by both colonic transit and defecatory alterations.

In order to allow the type of physiopathological mechanism to guide therapy, the most important diagnostic step is to establish whether the patient presents with slow colonic and/or rectal transit by studying large intestinal segmental transit time. To properly discriminate rectal from colonic slowing with radiopaque markers, it is useful to obtain a laterolateral radiograph when markers are located within the pelvic area on the anteroposterior radiograph [11] (fig. 1). On the basis of the findings of this examination, patients may present one of four pictures [12]: (1) normal intestinal transit; (2) colonic slowing; (3) rectal slowing; (4) rectocolonic slowing.

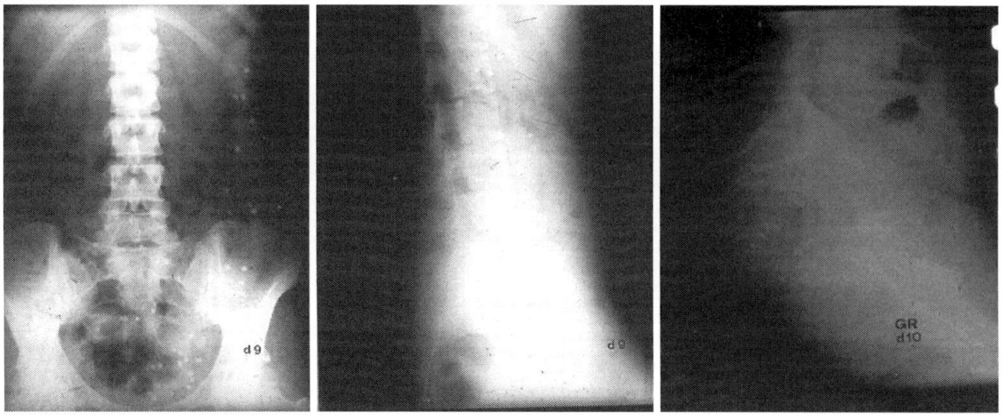

Fig. 1. Segmental colorectal transit time. Left and middle images are radiograms from the same patient obtained 9 days after ingestion of radiopaque markers. On the left anteroposterior radiogram, the radio-opaque markers are visible along the left colon and within the pelvis. The laterolateral radiogram obtained at the same time shows the gas-filled rectum without any markers indicating a slow colonic transit. The right laterolateral radiogram of another patient shows the markers retained in the rectum indicating slow rectal transit.

Furthermore, performing a transit study while the patient reports bowel movements on a diary offers valuable information on stool shape, frequency and modality of evacuation and their relationship with colorectal transit. To reinforce a patient's awareness of the origin of his/her disorder and thus increase treatment compliance, it is useful to describe to the patient his/her pattern of transit. In the case of normal transit accompanied by normal evacuations, they realize that they can evacuate completely without the need for any stimulus, and this is even more important in those whose continuous use of laxatives has led to them losing an awareness of their ability to have spontaneous bowel movements. In patients who deny evacuating, the finding of normal transit is an indication for psychiatric consultation.

Patients with Rectal Slowing or Normal Transit

Altered defecation in patients on a diet with an appropriate fiber content who do not present slow colonic transit or who are affected by rectal slowing is usually due to altered stool shape, size, and consistency, ano-recto-pelvic alterations and/or psychosocial disorders (fig. 2).

Under normal conditions, evacuation is the result of the coordinated contraction of the diaphragm and abdominal muscles, and appropriate pelvic floor inhibition triggered by the arrival of an adequate amount of feces in the rectum to evoke the stimulus to defecate. The presence of hard or pellet-shaped feces, impaired rectal sensitivity and/or a failure to relax (or the paradoxical contraction of) the outer anal sphincter and the puborectalis, and/or insufficient intraabdominal pressure during straining can variously alter the act of defecation.

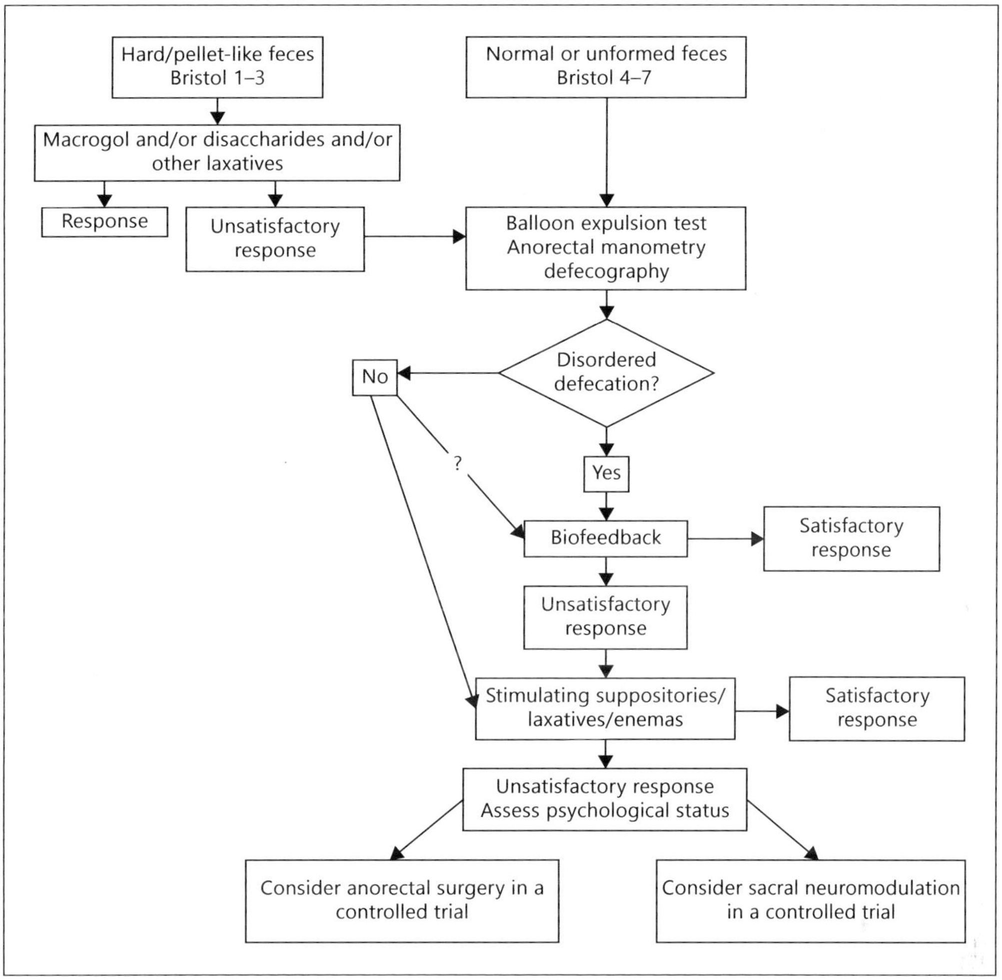

Fig. 2. Proposed diagnostic and therapeutic algorithm for patients with refractory constipation, normal transit or slow rectal transit.

Hard and small pellet-like feces are more difficult to evacuate because this requires considerable abdominal torque and leads to the insufficient emptying of the rectum. The use of macrogol or oral osmotic laxatives prevents fecal dehydration, softens or normalizes the feces, and significantly reduces the evacuative effort. One particular condition due to the accumulation of feces in the rectal ampulla is the formation of a fecaloma, which leads to distension of the walls and megarectum. This condition occurs mainly in infants [13] and the elderly, and the fecaloma must first be eliminated by means of a high dose of orally administered macrogol solution [14] or a hyperosmolar enema until the large intestine has been fully emptied; the efficacy of this procedure can be enhanced by the previous rectal administration of mineral oil.

Treatment is thereafter based on programmed evacuations and bowel reeducation by means of the regular use of laxatives and/or anorectal rehabilitation by means of bio-feedback (see below). In those who are incapable of cooperating, it may be advisable to administer daily doses of a laxative to soften the feces in order to prevent pain or difficulties when defecating.

Patients whose feces are normal or soft, and those who report the persistence of disordered evacuation after the consistency of their feces has been normalized by means of laxatives, should undergo further examinations aimed at revealing any functional disorders characterized by the finding of reduced rectal sensitivity or insufficient evacuation capacity due to a failure to inhibit the anopelvic musculature (abdominopelvic dyssynergia) or insufficient propulsion. The balloon expulsion test and anorectal manometry are risk-free and minimally invasive diagnostic examinations that are useful for evaluating defecatory function [1, 15]. More invasive electromyography of the pelvic floor is indicated when there is a suspicion of neuromyopathy. Traditional or nuclear magnetic resonance defecography makes it possible to evaluate the dynamics of defecation and any functional (abdominopelvic dyssynergia, anal canal opening and the degree of rectal emptying) or anatomical alterations (rectoceles, rectoanorectal intussusception, prolapse). For a complete review of anorectal tests, see Rao and Meduri [1].

No sign, symptom or test can per se diagnose the clinical relevance of any of the recto-ano-pelvic functional or structural alterations. In addition, there is no standard approach to, and different techniques have been used for, any single test. Finally, these tests have detected functional abnormalities in asymptomatic subjects and, not infrequently, yield opposite conclusions in the same patient. Hence, any test should be interpreted with clinical wisdom by properly trained experts along with other tests, and all relevant clinical clues.

Biofeedback and other physiotherapeutic techniques have proved to be efficacious in improving rectal sensitivity and the synergism between diaphragm-abdominal wall contraction and pelvic floor relaxation. Patients with reduced rectal sensitivity and functional defecatory disorders benefit from bowel reeducation and pelvic floor rehabilitation after normal fecal consistency has been restored. Such techniques have been reported to improve constipation in a large proportion of patients, although 15% do not respond and, among those who do, 14% continue to have recourse to digital evacuation and 11 and 85% continue to use high or low laxative doses, respectively [16, 17].

A meta-analysis suggested that biofeedback conferred a sixfold increase in the likelihood of symptomatic relief. Owing to the small number of trials, their heterogeneous nature and the lack of rigorous methodology, e.g. the lack of blinding, a definitive conclusion on the efficacy of biofeedback cannot be drawn [18]. Biofeedback is indicated in patients with pelvic dyssynergia, but having no risk of adverse events has been applied also in other types of constipation, regardless of the presence of alterations in defecation [19].

Patients not responding to anorectal-pelvic rehabilitation can be treated by means of twice- or thrice-weekly stimulation using suppositories, glycerine or bisacodyl, hyperosmolar, simple or medicated enemas (whichever is the least aggressive and has the least number of side effects at the same level of efficacy). Continuous recourse to enemas to stimulate evacuation is generally poorly tolerated in the long term, which suggests a need to consider surgery or sacral neuromodulation. However, before undertaking any invasive treatment subject to risks, a careful search should be made for any relevant psychological alterations.

Patients with Psychological Alterations

Patients with functional constipation are often affected by psychological disorders [20], and some studies indicate that depression can be considered an independent risk factor for constipation. More than 60% of constipated patients have one or more, frequently subthreshold, psychopathological disorders (most commonly anxiety and/or depression, followed by eating disorders, pain-related disorders) that generally precede the onset of constipation and, therefore, cannot always be interpreted as a reaction to the functional disorder. Furthermore, 40% of patients with psychiatric disorders are affected by primary or secondary constipation (mainly due to drug treatment). It is, therefore, always necessary to investigate the possible presence of psychological alterations in patients with chronic constipation, particularly if it is refractory. Personality, stress and the way in which they first learned to manage their bowel movements, all affect the way in which patients describe their intestinal disorders, the modality of evacuation, and their pathophysiogical recto-ano-pelvic alterations. Some patients may ignore the stimulus to defecate or deliberately repress evacuation by holding back their feces; others may report that they are suffering from constipation even when their frequency of evacuation is normal, and others with obsessive-compulsive behavior perform repetitive rituals of intestinal emptying because they are convinced that they are constipated. Stressful events have a considerable impact on the onset and course of chronic constipation: for example, a history of sexual and/or physical violence can have a significant effect on the severity of the (often refractory) clinical picture, and result in a lack of responsiveness to both conservative and surgical treatment [21]. The presence of psychobehavioral alterations, or a history of traumatic stress, should be suspected when a patient denies evacuating at all, when the symptoms are disproportionate to the objective findings of functional tests, and when the abdominal pain and bloating or defecatory disorders are continuous, unrelated to intestinal emptying, and do not improve despite treatment. The presence of gastrointestinal comorbidities such as gastroesophageal reflux disease or dyspepsia, or somatization disorders with extragastrointestinal comorbidities (often accompanied by fatigue, headache and irritability) are associated with, and should arouse suspicion of, psychopathological alterations [22].

Surgery

Surgical interventions should be performed in centers dedicated to the management of patients with refractory constipation, and the decision to proceed to surgery based on a joint evaluation of each case by a gastroenterologist, a colorectal surgeon, a psychiatrist, and any other appropriate specialist (such as a urologist, gynecologist or neurologist, depending on the presence of concomitant diseases). Because of the high risk of therapeutic failure, surgery is not indicated or should be considered very prudently in the case of patients whose prevalent disturbance is abdominal distension and/or pain, continuous pelvic pain, or other functional gastrointestinal or extra-gastrointestinal comorbidities, somatization disorders or serious psychological alterations.

Surgery may be considered in the case of patients with anatomical anorectal-pelvic alterations that do not respond satisfactorily to conservative treatment. Several surgical methods have been developed; however, their use depends more on the surgeon's preference than on scientific evidence.

Rectoceles or rectal intussusception are often present in patients with disordered defecation but, as they are also frequent in the general population, there are no standardized or objective criteria for assessing the pathogenetic role played by these anatomical alterations. Recommendations are largely based on only clinical judgments made from time to time in individual patients. Surgery can eliminate rectal intussusception or internal rectal relapse, correct rectoceles, and restore the anatomical continuity of the rectal wall. However, it is not possible to foresee the outcome in an individual patient because there are no criteria or diagnostic studies which can predict clinical outcome preoperatively; not surprisingly, an improvement in the bowel disorder is obtained in fewer than half of all operated patients [9]. Furthermore, surgery is not devoid of risk because of the large number of possible complications and their severity [23]. As many centers have applied these techniques without any evidence being acquired concerning their efficacy, experts in the field have declared that surgery should only be used in the context of controlled clinical trials carried out in reference centers with proven expertise in managing refractory constipation [24]. Respecting this practice has been made all the more necessary since a comparative study demonstrated the superiority of conservative macrogol treatment over stapled transanal rectal resection, and also confirmed the high risk of complications associated with the latter [10].

Sacral Neuromodulation

Previously successfully used to control anal incontinence, direct electrical stimulation of the sacral roots S2, S3 or S4 by means of electrodes has also been used with favorable results in the treatment of constipation. It is believed that its effect occurs as a result of the neuromodulation of the extrinsic nervous control (or intrinsic inhibitory reflexes) of the large intestine. The definitive surgical application of the electrodes to the sacral roots by means of the subcutaneous implantation of a stimulator only takes place after a positive response has been obtained to temporary, transcutaneously inserted, removable electrodes. In the absence of controlled studies, the evidence concerning the efficacy of this therapy is limited, but recourse to this technique performed in the context of a clinical trial conducted by a reference center can be considered in patients who fail to respond to conservative treatment. Unsatisfactory results have been reported in about 12% of cases. Dislocation of the electrodes is frequent, and pain and implant infections have been reported in 13 and 4% of cases, respectively [25, 26].

Conclusions

Considering difficult defecation simply a bowel alteration does not take into account the complexity of the clinical picture that usually develops in patients who fail to respond to initial therapy, which also involves the emotional and cognitive spheres by modifying behavior and affecting the patients' state of health. The various clinical expressions of the disorder (from mild to severe), and the limitations of the different treatments which, individually, do not guarantee a satisfactory resolution in 20–30% of patients, means that the most difficult cases require a further series of diagnostic investigations and therapeutic attempts in order to establish the optimal therapy.

References

1 Rao SSC, Meduri K: What is necessary to diagnose constipation? Best Pract Res Clin Gastroenterol 2011;25:127–140.
2 Shorvon PJ, Mc Hugh S, Diamant NE, et al: Defecography in normal volunteers: results and implications. Gut 1989;30:1737–1746.
3 Candeloro L, Badiali D, Cappuccio R, et al: Is there any difference in the defecographic detection of pelvic floor disorders between constipated and non constipated patients? Dig Liv Dis 2009;415:598–599.
4 Johanson JF, Sonnenberg A: Constipation is not a risk factor for hemorrhoids: a case control study of potential etiological agents. Am J Gastroenterol 1994;89:1981–1986.
5 Pigot F, Siproudhis L, Allaert FA: Risk factors associated with hemorrhoidal symptoms in specialized consultation. Gastroenterol Clin Biol 2005;29:1270–1274.
6 Morio O, Meurette G, Desfourneaux V, D'Halluin PN, Bretagne JF, Siproudhis L: Anorectal physiology in solitary ulcer syndrome: a case matched series. Dis Colon Rect 2005;48:1917–1922.
7 Bulut T, Canbay E, Yamaner S, Gulluoglu M, Bugra D: Solitary rectal ulcer syndrome: exploring possible management options. Int Surg 2011;96:45–50.
8 Maurer CA, Renzulli P, Mazzucchelli L, Egger B, Seiler CA, Büchler MW: Use of accurate diagnostic criteria may increase incidence of stercoral perforation of the colon. Dis Colon Rectum 2000;43:991–998.
9 Drossman DA, Corazziari E, Delvaux M, et al: Functional Gastrointestinal Disorders. ROME III 2006. McLean, Degnon Associates, 2006.
10 Biviano I, Badiali D, Candeloro L, et al: Comparative outcome of stapled trans-anal rectal resection and macrogol in the treatment of defecation disorders. World J Gastroenterol 2011;17:4199–4205.
11 Corazziari E, Dani S, Pozzessere C, Anzini F, Torsoli A: Colonic segmental transit time in non-organic constipation. Rendic Gastroenterol 1975;7:65–69.

12 Menardo G, Bausano G, Corazziari E, et al: Large bowel transit in paraplegic patients. Dis Colon Rectum 1987;30:924–928.

13 Cucchiara S, Coremans G, Staiano A, et al: Gastrointestinal transit time and anorectal manometry in children with fecal soiling. J Pediatr Gastroenterol Nutr 1984;3:545–550.

14 Ferguson A, Culbert H, Gillet H, Barras N: New PEG/electrolyte solution for the treatment of constipation and fecal impaction. Ital J Gastroenterol Hepatol 1999;31(suppl 3):S249–S252.

15 Bharucha AE, Wald A, Enck P, Rao S: Functional anorectal disorders. Gastroenterology 2006;130: 1510–1518.

16 Rao SS, Welcher KD, Pelsang RE: Effects of biofeedback therapy on anorectal function in obstructive defecation. Dig Dis Sci 1977;42:2197–2205.

17 Chiarioni G, Whitehead WE, Pezza V, Morelli A, Bassotti G: Biofeedback is superior to laxatives for normal transit constipation due to pelvic floor dyssynergia. Gastroenterology 2006;130:657–664.

18 Koh CE, Young CJ, Young JM, Solomon MJ: Systematic review of randomized controlled trials of the effectiveness of biofeedback for pelvic floor dysfunction Br J Surg 2008;95:1079–1087.

19 Chiotakakou-Faliakou E, Kamm MA, Roy AJ, Storrie JB, Turner I: Biofeedback provides long-term benefit for patients with intractable, slow and normal transit constipation. Gut 1998;42:517–521.

20 Levy RL, Olden KW, Naliboff BD, et al: Psychosocial aspects of the functional gastrointestinal disorders. Gastroenterology 2006;130:1447–1458.

21 O'Brien S, Hyman N, Osler T, Rabinowitz T: Sexual abuse: a strong predictor of outcomes after colectomy for slow transit constipation. Dis Colon Rectum 2009;152:1844–1847.

22 Piacentino D, Cantarini R, Alfonsi M, et al: Psychopathological features of irritable bowel syndrome patients with and without functional dyspepsia: a cross sectional study. BMC Gastroenterol 2011;11:94.

23 Dodi G, Pietroletti R, Milito G, Binda G, Pescatori M: Bleeding, incontinence, pain and constipation after STARR transanal double stapling rectotomy for obstructed defecation. Tech Coloproctol 2003;7:148–153.

24 Corman ML, Carriero A, Hager T, et al: Consensus conference on the stapled transanal rectal resection (STARR) for disordered defaecation. Colorectal Dis 2006;8:98–101.

25 Maeda Y, Matzel K, Lundby L, Buntzen S, Laurberg S: Postoperative issues of sacral nerve stimulation for fecal incontinence and constipation: a systematic literature review and treatment guideline. Dis Colon Rectum 2011;54:1443–1460.

26 van Wunnik BP, Baeten CG, Southwell BR: Neuromodulation for constipation: sacral and transcutaneous stimulation. Best Pract Res Clin Gastroenterol 2011;25:181–191.

Enrico Stefano Corazziari
Dipartimento di Medicina Interna e Specialità Mediche, Università Sapienza ROMA
V.le del Policlinico Umberto I, 155
IT–00161 Roma (Italy)
E-Mail enrico.corazziari@uniroma1.it

Quigley EMM, Hongo M, Fukudo S (eds): Functional and GI Motility Disorders.
Front Gastrointest Res. Basel, Karger, 2014, vol 33, pp 95–103 (DOI: 10.1159/000356783)

Functional Gastrointestinal Disorders: The Mind-Body Dimension

Lukas Van Oudenhove

Translational Research Center for Gastrointestinal Disorders (TARGID), Department of Clinical and Experimental Medicine, University of Leuven, and University Psychiatric Centre Campus Gasthuisberg, Liaison Psychiatry, Leuven, Belgium

Abstract

This chapter will focus on the growing body of evidence identifying the biological basis of mind-body interactions which may explain the role of psychosocial factors and psychiatric disorders in functional gastrointestinal disorders (FGID). First, a model of FGID as disorders of gut-brain signaling will be outlined, illustrating the principal (patho)physiological mechanisms of brain processing of visceral sensory signals in a homeostatic-afferent network, which is subject to modulation by emotional-arousal and cortical-modulatory regions through the descending modulatory system. Second, recent evidence, mainly from functional brain imaging studies, will be discussed, supporting substantial cognitive and affective modulation of homeostatic-afferent signals in healthy subjects as well as a key pathophysiological role of these mechanisms in FGID, as postulated in the model. I will emphasize similar findings in irritable bowel syndrome and functional dyspepsia research, despite methodological differences between studies. Abnormalities in activity and connectivity of emotional-arousal and cortical-modulatory circuits involved in pain modulation, which may lead to increased activity in homeostatic-afferent pain-processing regions through failing descending modulation, have indeed been shown to underlie the heightened anticipatory anxiety and increased perceptual sensitivity for visceral sensations in both of these disorders. This may help identify multidimensional endophenotypes, taking into account a combination of psychological and neurophysiological mechanisms, which may not be specific to a single FGID, but indeed common to (visceral) pain disorders in general. These may be crucial to make progress in the understanding of the pathophysiology of complex, heterogeneous, symptom-based disorders such as FGID, which may help identify more homogeneous subgroups and ultimately treatments that are better tailored to the individual patient.

Functional gastrointestinal disorders (FGID) are characterized by chronic, bothersome abdominal symptoms, including visceral pain, that cannot readily be explained by organic causes. Recent epidemiological evidence confirms an important intrinsic role for psychological processes and psychiatric comorbidity, most notably mood and anxiety disorders, in the etiopathogenesis of FGID. A meta-analysis published in 2003 clearly demonstrated a significant association with mood and anxiety disorders for both irritable bowel syndrome (IBS), the prototypical functional bowel disorder, and functional dyspepsia (FD), the most prevalent functional disorder of the upper gastrointestinal (GI) tract [1]. More recent studies have confirmed this association and extended it to population-based rather than consulting samples, indicating that psychological morbidity may play a central role in FGID etiopathogenesis, rather than merely driving health care seeking in these patients. However, excellent recent reviews focusing on epidemiological aspects of the association between psychosocial factors, psychiatric disorders and FGID are available [2, 3], and this will also be covered in another chapter in this book [4]. Therefore, in this chapter I will focus on the growing body of evidence identifying the biological basis of mind-body interactions which may explain the role of psychosocial factors and psychiatric disorders in FGID. First, I will outline a model of FGID as disorders of gut-brain signaling. Second, I will discuss recent evidence, mainly from functional brain imaging studies, supporting a critical role for cognitive and affective modulation of homeostatic-afferent signals in FGID, as postulated in the model. I will emphasize similar findings in IBS and FD research, despite methodological differences between studies. This may help identify multidimensional endophenotypes, taking into account a combination of psychological and neurophysiological mechanisms, which may not be specific to a single FGID, but indeed common to (visceral) pain disorders in general.

Model of Functional Gastrointestinal Disorders as Disorders of Gut-Brain Signaling

The 'brain-gut axis', the bidirectional neurohumoral communication system between the brain and the gut, is integrated into the interoceptive system which is continuously signaling homeostatic information about the physiological condition of the body to the brain [for an excellent review on this topic, see 5]. Under normal physiological circumstances, the vast majority of the continuous stream of interoceptive gut-brain signals remains outside conscious awareness. However, the unpleasant subjective experience of visceral pain results from the conscious perception of gut-brain signaling induced by noxious stimuli, indicating potential threat to homeostasis and potentially requiring a behavioral response (fig. 1a). At the brain level, visceral pain-related interoceptive signals are processed in a homeostatic-afferent network (brainstem sensory nuclei including the nucleus of the solitary tract and the parabrachial nucleus, thalamus, posterior insula) and integrated with and modulated by emotional-arousal [locus coeruleus in the dorsal pons, amygdala, subgenual anterior cingulate cortex (sACC)] and cortical-modulatory [prefrontal cortex (PFC) subregions, anterior insula, perigenual ACC (pACC)] neurocircuits.

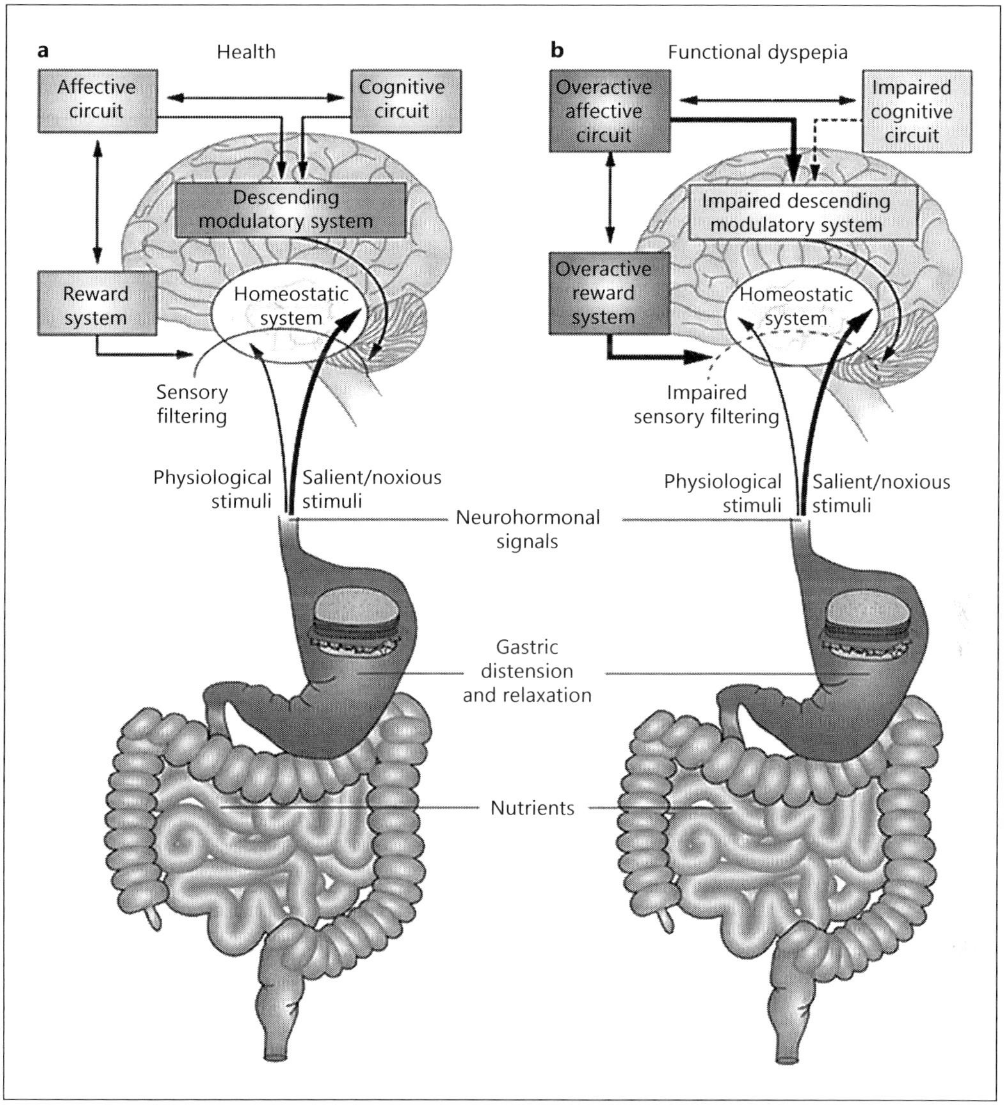

Fig. 1. Model of functional dyspepsia as a disorder of gut-brain signaling. **a** The presence of food in the GI tract is signaled to homeostatic regions in the brain via neurohormonal pathways. This signaling is largely unperceived, with only salient or potentially noxious stimuli requiring a behavioral response reaching consciousness owing to a sensory filtering process that involves the reward system and 'top-down' projections from affective and cognitive circuits (descending modulatory system). **b** Normal sensory signaling from the GI tract to the brain might be inappropriately perceived in the case of defective sensory filtering, for instance in the case of an overactive reward system or an impaired descending modulatory system, which might be related to psychological processes such as anxiety (overactive affective circuit) or impaired cognitive inhibition. This defective sensory filtering might impair food intake regulation as well as increase perception of physiological stimuli as painful. This model takes functional dyspepsia as an example, but is equally applicable to other functional GI disorders including IBS. Reproduced with permission from Van Oudenhove and Aziz [3].

Key regions in these emotional-arousal and cortical-modulatory circuits project in a 'top-down' fashion to brainstem areas such as the periaqueductal gray and the rostral ventrolateral medulla, which in turn send descending projections to the dorsal horn of the spinal cord, where pain transmission is modulated *(descending modulatory system)*. This circuitry forms the biological basis of cognitive and emotional modulation of (visceral) pain (see below). Dysfunction of this modulatory system may allow physiological (non-noxious) stimuli to be perceived as painful or unpleasant *(hypersensitivity)*, which may lead to chronic visceral pain and/or discomfort, hallmarks of most FGID (fig. 1b) [6–9]. This model is crucial to understand the biological basis of how psychosocial factors and psychiatric disorders may influence (functional) GI symptoms in general and visceral pain as a hallmark symptom of FGID in particular. Empirical functional brain imaging evidence supporting this model will be outlined below, emphasizing similar mechanisms in IBS and FD, after discussing some relevant findings on how psychological processes may modulate (visceral) pain in healthy subjects.

Psychological Modulation of Visceral Pain in Healthy Subjects

Emotional Modulation

A relatively large body of experimental as well as clinical evidence suggests that negative and positive emotional states may increase and decrease somatic pain perception, respectively [10], and we are starting to unravel the brain mechanisms underlying this emotional modulation of pain [11]. However, evidence for emotional modulation of visceral pain, although assumed to play a critical role in visceral pain disorders including FGID (see previous paragraph), is relatively sparse. Coen et al. [12] demonstrated that negative emotion induction (using validated classical music pieces) increased the brain response to painful esophageal stimulation in key pain-processing (homeostatic-afferent) brain regions, including mid-cingulate cortex and insula, as well as in a modulatory region (ventrolateral PFC), compared to neutral emotion induction. However, contrary to its effect on brain responses, negative emotion induction did not increase subjective responses (i.e. pain ratings) to the esophageal stimulation, which may be due to the fact that the study was powered for detecting differences in brain responses, and not for detecting rather subtle effects on subjective responses. A large recent study (n = 80), however, clearly demonstrated an increase and decrease in subjective ratings of identical esophageal pain stimuli during negative and positive emotion induction, respectively, using a combination of classical music pieces, affective pictures and emotional statements [Weltens et al., unpubl. data]. However, interindividual variability in emotional modulation of pain is large, and the psychobiological mechanisms underlying this variability remain to be identified.

Cognitive Modulation

Similar to emotional modulation, the influence of various cognitive processes, especially attention/distraction, on somatic pain is well known, and knowledge of the underlying brain processes is gradually increasing [13]. Less is known about visceral pain, but Coen et al. [14] showed that distraction was associated with a significant reduction in pain ratings accompanied by a reduction of activity in the ACC and PFC subregions. This physiological phenomenon may help us understand the putative influence of hypervigilance for visceral stimuli on pain perception in FGID patients.

Psychobiological Mechanisms in Functional Gastrointestinal Disorders: Evidence from Functional Brain Imaging Studies

Brain Activity

FD patients are characterized by activation of homeostatic-afferent brain regions (for example the insula and somatosensory cortex) at lower intragastric pressures than healthy controls, as shown using $H_2{}^{15}O$-positron emission tomography (PET) [15]. This may represent the neural basis of the observation that FD patients perceive gastric distension as unpleasant or painful at substantially lower intragastric pressures than healthy individuals (that is, hypersensitivity to gastric distension) [16]. Moreover, during painful gastric distension, patients with FD fail to activate the pACC, a key region in the descending modulatory system, and fail to deactivate the locus coeruleus, a noradrenergic brainstem nucleus that is a key node of the modulatory emotional-arousal circuit. Further, increased anxiety levels correlate significantly with lower pACC and higher locus coeruleus activity in FD. Finally, during anticipated gastric distension, patients fail to deactivate the amygdala, another key emotional-arousal region [15].

Despite methodological differences, remarkably similar findings are reported in IBS. A meta-analysis of functional brain imaging studies demonstrated more activation of homeostatic-afferent (insula, mid-cingulate cortex, thalamus) and emotional arousal (amygdala) regions in IBS patients versus controls, whereas the healthy controls were characterized by more activation in prefrontal cortical-modulatory regions [17]. Berman et al. [18] used functional magnetic resonance imaging and fixed stimulus intensity rectal distensions (as opposed to the individually titrated painful distensions used in the FD study mentioned above) to study brain responses to rectal pain and its anticipation in IBS. First, more extensive activation of the insula, the key homeostatic-afferent brain region, was found in IBS patients compared to controls during rectal distension at the same stimulus intensity, which may again represent the rectal hypersensitivity observed in IBS patients. Further, hyperactivation of the locus coeruleus was found in IBS patients compared to controls, which is in line with the lack of deactivation of this emotional arousal region observed in FD. Moreover, as in FD, anxiety levels correlated positively with locus coeruleus activity, which in turn correlated negatively with pACC activity in IBS patients. Finally, similar to FD, deactivation of the amygdala during anticipation of distension was found in healthy controls, but not IBS patients. Another study by Berman et al. [19] used a combination of a pharmacological challenge with the α_2-adrenoreceptor antagonist yohimbine and PET imaging to further elucidate the role of the noradrenaline in the abnormalities in emotional arousal circuit function found in IBS patients versus controls. Patients had higher noradrenaline levels at baseline, and yohimbine had a significantly higher effect on noradrenaline and anxiety levels compared to controls. This was accompanied by less yohimbine-induced reduction of activity in key emotional-arousal regions including the locus coeruleus, amygdala and sACC in IBS patients, consistent with less functional α_2-receptors dampening activity in the emotional-arousal circuit. A history of trauma was also associated with less yohimbine-induced reduction of activity in similar regions, highlighting the important influence of trauma on the function of the emotional-arousal circuit, which was also found in FD [20]. A more recent study by the same UCLA group confirmed an increased locus coeruleus response to abdominal pain threat in IBS patients compared to healthy controls, and demonstrated that this response could be normalized by pretreatment with a corticotropin-releasing factor-1 receptor (CRF_1R) antagonist, identifying the CRF system as a key neurotransmitter involved in the pathophysiology of IBS through its influence on the regulation of emotional-arousal circuitry [21]. Further, a single nucleotide polymorphism in the serotonin-3 receptor ($5\text{-}HT_3R$) gene (CC > T) was shown to be associated with both higher anxiety and increased amygdala activity in an affect-matching paradigm, thereby elucidating the genetic underpinnings of the abnormal amygdala reactivity observed in both FD and IBS patients [22].

Brain Connectivity

Besides the studies reporting on differences in brain activity in response to (anticipation of) visceral pain outlined in the paragraph above, more recent studies focused on differences in connectivity within homeostatic-afferent, emotional-arousal and cortical-modulatory circuitry between FGID patients and controls.

In FD patients, altered connectivity in homeostatic-afferent, emotional-arousal and cortical-modulatory circuitry underlies the increased perceptual sensitivity for gastric sensation compared to healthy controls [23]. These abnormalities include altered 'bottom-up' signaling from emotional-arousal regions, particularly the locus coeruleus and the sACC to the pACC, which is in turn defectively connected to the periaqueductal gray, a key pathway of the descending modulatory system ('top-down'). During anticipation, a lack of negative connectivity from the pACC to the amygdala was observed as well. Further, within the FD patients, those with a history of severe sexual or physical abuse are characterized by increased perceptual sensitivity for gastric sensation compared to those without such a history, and this is related to differences in connectivity in emotional-arousal (selective attention to threat) and cortical-modulatory circuits, particularly impaired 'top-down' connectivity to the amygdala [20].

In IBS, again, fairly similar findings have been reported despite some methodological differences between the studies. First, Labus et al. [24] found impaired 'top-down' connectivity to the amygdala within the emotional-arousal circuit in IBS patients compared to healthy controls. Interestingly, the connectivity pattern found in IBS could be mimicked in healthy controls by using acute tryptophan depletion, which temporarily decreases serotonin levels. This points towards an important role for the serotonin neurotransmitter system in explaining abnormalities in emotional-arousal circuit connectivity which may underlie anxiety, hypervigilance for interoceptive stimuli and increased perceptual sensitivity for visceral sensations in IBS. In the study by Hubbard et al. [21] already mentioned above, administration of a selective CRF_1 receptor antagonist was shown to normalize effective connectivity in the emotional-arousal circuit in IBS patients, with less pronounced effects observed in healthy controls.

Towards Psychophysiological Endophenotypes in Functional Gastrointestinal Disorders?

Taken together, this emerging evidence from functional brain imaging is gradually unraveling the biological mechanisms underlying the phenomena of emotional and cognitive modulation of pain, which may explain the link between psychological processes, psychiatric comorbidity and symptom generation in FGID, including FD and IBS. As FGID are syndromes which are currently defined purely based on symptom criteria, they inherently have a heterogeneous pathophysiology, which is multifactorial and biopsychosocial in nature. Therefore, one single pathophysiological mechanism or biomarker is very unlikely to explain FGID symptoms. Thus, an integrative approach is needed where the complex interaction of different potentially relevant pathophysiological processes is taken into account, including psychological processes, psychiatric comorbidity and their neurobiological underpinnings. Such an approach may ultimately lead to the identification of 'endophenotypes' defined as 'measurable components unseen by the unaided eye along the pathway between disease phenotype and distal genotype' [25]. Endophenotypes may be especially relevant in symptom-based disorders or syndromes such as psychiatric disorders and FGID, as the mechanisms underlying their phenotype are heterogeneous. Moreover, endophenotypes can be of various and multidimensional nature, including biochemical, neurophysiological and (neuro)psychological aspects. Further, endophenotypes are not necessarily syndrome-specific and may indeed be shared by different symptom-based disorders. Based on the emerging evidence from functional brain imaging studies in IBS and FD outlined in this chapter, abnormal activity and connectivity in emotional-arousal circuitry interfering with descending modulatory pathways, manifesting itself clinically as increased (symptom-specific) anxiety and hypervigilance to bodily signals and perceptual hypersensitivity for visceral sensations, may serve as a candidate endophenotype that may not be specific to one but indeed common to all FGID or even other (visceral) pain disorders. Moreover, we are starting to identify neurotransmitter systems involved in the (dys)function of these brain circuits through pharmacologic and genetic brain imaging approaches.

References

1 Henningsen P, Zimmermann T, Sattel H: Medically unexplained physical symptoms, anxiety, and depression: a meta-analytic review. Psychosom Med 2003;65:528–533.

2 Surdea Blaga T, Baban A, Dumitrascu D: Psychosocial determinants of irritable bowel syndrome. World J Gastroenterol 2012;18:616–626.

3 Van Oudenhove L, Aziz Q: The role of psychosocial factors and psychiatric disorders in functional dyspepsia. Nat Rev Gastroenterol Hepatol 2013;10:158–167.

4 Lackner JM: Psychosocial aspects of functional gastrointestinal disorders; in Quigley EMM, Hongo M, Fukudo S (eds): Functional and GI Motility Disorders. Front Gastrointest Res. Basel, Karger, 2013, vol 33, pp 104–116.

5 Mayer EA: Gut feelings: the emerging biology of gut-brain communication. Nat Rev Neurosci 2011;12:453–466.

6 Fields H: State-dependent opioid control of pain. Nat Rev Neurosci 2004;5:565–575.

7 Wilder-Smith CH: The balancing act: endogenous modulation of pain in functional gastrointestinal disorders. Gut 2011;60:1589–1599.

8 Mayer EA, Naliboff BD, Craig ADB: Neuroimaging of the brain-gut axis: from basic understanding to treatment of functional GI disorders. Gastroenterology 2006;131:1925–1942.

9 Van Oudenhove L: Understanding gut-brain interactions in gastrointestinal pain by neuroimaging: lessons from somatic pain studies. Neurogastroenterol Motil 2011;23:292–302.

10 Klossika I, Flor H, Kamping S, Bleichhardt G, Trautmann N, Treede R-D, Bohus M, Schmahl C: Emotional modulation of pain: a clinical perspective. Pain 2006;124:264–268.

11 Wiech K, Tracey I: The influence of negative emotions on pain: behavioral effects and neural mechanisms. Neuroimage 2009;47:987–994.

12 Coen SJ, Yágüez L, Aziz Q, Mitterschiffthaler MT, Brammer M, Williams SCR, Gregory LJ: Negative mood affects brain processing of visceral sensation. Gastroenterology 2009;137:253–261.

13 Wiech K, Ploner M, Tracey I: Neurocognitive aspects of pain perception. Trends Cogn Sci 2008;12:306–313.

14 Coen SJ, Aziz Q, Yagüez L, Brammer M, Williams SCR, Gregory LJ: Effects of attention on visceral stimulus intensity encoding in the male human brain. Gastroenterology 2008;135:2065–2074.

15 Van Oudenhove L, Vandenberghe J, Dupont P, Geeraerts B, Vos R, Dirix S, Van Laere K, Bormans G, Vanderghinste D, Demyttenaere K, Fischler B, Tack J: Abnormal regional brain activity during rest and (anticipated) gastric distension in functional dyspepsia and the role of anxiety: a $H_2{}^{15}O$-PET study. Am J Gastroenterol 2010;105:913–924.

16 Tack J, Caenepeel P, Fischler B, Piessevaux H, Janssens J: Symptoms associated with hypersensitivity to gastric distention in functional dyspepsia. Gastroenterology 2001;121:526–535.

17 Tillisch K, Mayer EA, Labus JS: Quantitative meta-analysis identifies brain regions activated during rectal distension in irritable bowel syndrome. Gastroenterology 2011;140:91–100.

18 Berman SM, Naliboff BD, Suyenobu B, Labus JS, Stains J, Ohning G, Kilpatrick L, Bueller JA, Ruby K, Jarcho J, Mayer EA: Reduced brainstem inhibition during anticipated pelvic visceral pain correlates with enhanced brain response to the visceral stimulus in women with irritable bowel syndrome. J Neurosci 2008;28:349–359.

19 Berman S, Suyenobu B, Naliboff BD, Bueller J, Stains J, Wong H, Mandelkern M, Fitzgerald L, Ohning G, Gupta A, Labus JS, Tillisch K, Mayer EA: Evidence for alterations in central noradrenergic signaling in irritable bowel syndrome. Neuroimage 2012;63:1854–1863.

20 Van Oudenhove L, Labus JS, Dupont P, Vandenberghe JU, Bormans G, Laere KV, Mayer EA, Tack JF: Altered brain connectivity underlies visceral perceptual hypersensitivity in abused functional dyspepsia patients. Gastroenterology 2012;142:S-69–S-70.
21 Hubbard CS, Labus JS, Bueller J, Stains J, Suyenobu B, Dukes GE, Kelleher DL, Tillisch K, Naliboff BD, Mayer EA: Corticotropin-releasing factor receptor 1 antagonist alters regional activation and effective connectivity in an emotional-arousal circuit during expectation of abdominal pain. J Neurosci 2011;31:12491–12500.
22 Kilpatrick LA, Labus JS, Coveleskie K, Hammer C, Rappold G, Tillisch K, Bueller JA, Suyenobu B, Jarcho JM, McRoberts JA, Niesler B, Mayer EA: The HTR3A polymorphism c. -42c>T is associated with amygdala responsiveness in patients with irritable bowel syndrome. Gastroenterology 2011;140:1943–1951.
23 Van Oudenhove L, Labus J, Dupont P, Vandenberghe J, Vos R, Bormans G, Van Laere K, Demyttenaere K, Mayer E, Tack J: Altered brain network connectivity associated with increased perceptual response to aversive gastric distension and its expectation in functional dyspepsia. Neurogastroenterol Motil 2010;22:20–21.
24 Labus JS, Mayer EA, Jarcho J, Kilpatrick LA, Kilkens TOC, Evers EAT, Backes WH, Brummer R-JM, van Nieuwenhoven MA: Acute tryptophan depletion alters the effective connectivity of emotional arousal circuitry during visceral stimuli in healthy women. Gut 2011;60:1196–1203.
25 Gottesman II, Gould TD: The endophenotype concept in psychiatry: etymology and strategic intentions. Am J Psychiatry 2003;160:636–645.

Lukas Van Oudenhove
Translational Research Centre for Gastrointestinal Disorders (TARGID)
Herestraat 49, O&N I, Box 701
BE–3000 Leuven (Belgium)
E-Mail lukas.vanoudenhove@med.kuleuven.be

Quigley EMM, Hongo M, Fukudo S (eds): Functional and GI Motility Disorders.
Front Gastrointest Res. Basel, Karger, 2014, vol 33, pp 104–116 (DOI: 10.1159/000356785)

The Role of Psychosocial Factors in Functional Gastrointestinal Disorders

Jeffrey M. Lackner

Division of Gastroenterology, Department of Medicine, University at Buffalo School of Medicine, SUNY, Buffalo, N.Y., USA

Abstract

Lacking a biomarker that reliably corresponds with GI symptoms, functional GI disorders (FGIDs) are best understood from the perspective of a biopsychosocial model that emphasizes the reciprocal and interactive relationship among biological, environmental, and psychological factors. In more severe patients, psychological factors exert a particularly strong influence on the expression of GI symptoms and related distress. This chapter describes 3 different pathways that link psychological processes to FGIDs with a focus on irritable bowel syndrome: psychological processes as vulnerability factors (early life adversity, neuroticism, observational learning) that increase the risk of developing FGIDs; psychological factors as determinants of illness behaviors that aggravate the day-to-day burden of FGIDs; psychological factors that directly impact biological processes (e.g. motility) that influence core symptoms of FGIDs, and psychological processes that, if targeted through evidence-based treatments (e.g. cognitive behavior therapy), have potential to relieve physical symptoms of FGIDs unresponsive to conventional medical or dietary treatments for more severely affected patients. This paper will describe these pathways with a focus on the FGIDs about which most is known (irritable bowel syndrome).

Epidemiological data suggest that functional gastrointestinal disorders (FGIDs) are common and oftentimes disabling [1]. Irritable bowel syndrome (IBS) – the most common of FGIDs – affects 15% of the world's population at any given time. The addition of functional dyspepsia, chronic constipation, gastroesophageal reflux disease, and noncardiac chest pain makes FGIDs a public health problem of staggering proportions. Even though a small proportion of individuals with FGIDs seek medical care [2, 3], they account for 40–60% of all outpatient visits to GI clinics. Because they have no known etiology and their symptoms oftentimes mimic those of 'organic' diseases with underlying physical pathology, FGIDs are a source of frustration for physicians and of despair for patients, their families, and friends. Moreover, the costs –

direct and indirect – associated with FGIDs impose a significant burden on our health care systems.

Lacking a reliable biomarker, FGIDs are therefore best understood from a biopsychosocial perspective [4]. The biopsychosocial model of FGIDs holds that individual biology (e.g. genetic predisposition, GI physiology), behavior, and higher-order cognitive processes (e.g. coping, illness beliefs, abnormal central processing of gut stimuli) influence FGIDs through their interaction with each other, with early-life factors (e.g. trauma, negative learning experiences), and with the individual's social and physical environments (e.g. reinforcement contingencies, interpersonal stress). At the heart of the model is recognition that FGIDs involve a dysregulation in interactions among the cognitive and emotional centers of the central nervous system (CNS), the immune system, the neuroendocrine system, and the enteric nervous system. Although alterations at any level of the neuroenteric axis may result in hallmark features of symptoms of FGIDs, multiple lines of evidence underscore the importance of CNS activity in modulating symptoms, particularly in more severely affected patients seen in tertiary care settings. Research has pointed to four main pathways through which psychological factors influence GI symptoms of FGIDs. This chapter will describe these pathways with a focus on the FGIDs about which most is known (IBS). An excellent source of information regarding psychosocial factors associated with functional dyspepsia can be found elsewhere [5].

Psychological Factors Shape Physiological Responses

The first key pathway linking psychological factors and FGIDs is directly through physiological systems that mediate gut sensation and function. A full review of these data is beyond the scope of this chapter, but the reader is encouraged to refer to Chang [6] for an excellent review of the literature. One of the earliest and most dramatic examples comes from Almy and colleagues whose laboratory studies in the 1940s and 1950s were designed to clarify the impact of stress on colonic function. In one study (1951), a healthy, 22-year-old medical student underwent a protoscopy which presumably detected 'carcinoma of the rectum'. The investigators requested the student to sign a consent permitting them to perform a biopsy. During the period when the biopsy was presumably performed, the student demonstrated heightened reactivity of gut function as measured by vascular engorgement of the bowel and increased contractions of gut above and beyond what was observed during a 10-min baseline period. After the student was debriefed and informed that information about the discovery of carcinoma was a hoax, colonic motility and engorgement were reevaluated and found to return to baseline levels. In other words, gut reactivity corresponded with the presentation (and termination) of psychological stress. These data led Almy to conclude that the colonic response depends not only upon the stimulus but also upon the subject's interpretation of the stimulus [7].

While stress-induced change in GI function is universal across both healthy individuals and functional GI patients, they are exaggerated in patients with FGIDs on core pathophysiological dimensions (e.g. gut motility, visceral perception) [8, 9]. In one study linking laboratory induction of negative mood to increased colonic motility [8], IBS patients and controls underwent ambulatory motility recordings in the colon. Individuals in both groups were confronted on their return to the lab ('you're late', 'you came to the wrong window', 'now the study may need to be repeated') in a hostile manner that was designed to induce stress reactivity. Colonic motility increased during confrontation in the IBS patients, but not in healthy volunteers. A variety of psychological stressors (e.g. dichotomous listening tasks, driving in traffic, balls sorting) can elicit similar changes in GI motor function.

With respect to the effect of stress on visceral perception, there is some evidence that IBS patients report enhanced perceptual sensitivity when exposed to psychological stressors in laboratory settings. Dickhaus et al. [10], for example, reported that IBS patients reported significantly higher ratings of pain sensation and unpleasantness than controls following a rectal distension task while undergoing a psychologically stressful dichotomous listening tasks (i.e. different auditory inputs are played into the subjects' ears than controls). Similar findings have been reported by other researchers who have found that pain ratings fluctuate with the presentation of laboratory-induced psychological challenge [e.g. 11]. Other researchers have failed to find an effect of acute laboratory stressors on perception of colorectal distension. Inconsistent findings may be due to methodological differences in the design of studies. Even so, the picture that emerges from broad review of data is that psychological factors (e.g. stress, strong negative emotions) directly affect physiological systems underlying gut sensation and function. These conclusions dovetail with what IBS patients report about the relationship between stress and GI symptoms. IBS patients report that psychological stress more frequently affects pain and bowel patterns than control subjects. Further, IBS patients report more stressful events, more stress-related changes in stool patterns, and greater reactivity to stress than controls [12]. Creed et al. [13] found that major life events preceded the onset of IBS in 60–66% of IBS patients.

Psychological Factors Influence Illness Behaviors

A second pathway through which psychological factors influence IBS symptoms is the adoption of illness behaviors. The term 'illness behaviors' refers to maladaptive ways of responding to one's illness [14]. Illness behaviors can take one of two extreme forms [15]. At one end, an individual may fail to detect and act on troublesome somatic sensations that are amenable to medical treatment. An example is an elderly individual who does not seek appropriate care for chronic constipation because of the mistaken belief that it is a normative and uncontrollable part of the aging process for which there are no helpful treatments. At the other extreme are individuals who are preoccupied with fears of having a serious disease based on the person's interpretation of body sensations. These fears are behaviorally expressed in various forms such as resting in bed, taking excessive medications, urging doctors to perform diagnostic tests of limited value, 'doctor shopping', exhibiting facial expression of discomfort or verbal complaints, or engaging in avoidance behaviors. The most overt forms of avoidance include refusal to enter situations where symptoms are expected to occur (e.g. avoiding shopping in shopping malls where the location of bathrooms is unknown) and escaping from unpleasant situations shortly after entering (e.g. leaving a party after 15 min because of fear that low level of nausea will worsen and cause a loss of control).

In addition to overt behaviors, FGID patients can engage in more subtle 'safety behaviors' that are used to protect themselves from feeling overly uncomfortable or to prevent their undesirable consequences (e.g. loss of bowel control, embarrassment, pain) from actually occurring. Patients who engage in safety behaviors do not necessarily outright avoid a situation or activities but will only do so if they take certain precautions. For example, someone who is fearful of losing control of bowel function may only feel comfortable going out to dinner if she carries a bottle of Imodium or an extra pair of underwear in her purse. In this case, the bottle of Imodium becomes a 'safety signal'. Safety signals are regarded as more subtle forms of avoidance because they are believed to help the person escape or avoid a negative outcome. The individual assumes that managing symptoms depends on the safety signal, and the aversive situation is manageable only when the safety signal is present. Safety behaviors reinforce the assumption that the situation would be intolerable if the safety signal was absent. Engaging in safety behaviors prevents disconfirmation of threat appraisals, thereby heightening anxiety which can aggravate somatic symptoms. In the long term, excessive use of safety behaviors increases anxiety and self-focused attention and causes a misattribution of safety. That is, the patient who relies on safety behaviors to cope with IBS flare-ups attributes their nonoccurrence to a safety behavior not to his/her own coping behavior.

Patient Beliefs

Illness behaviors are influenced by how patients describe aspects of their illness. Patients vary in how they interpret their symptoms as well as the intensity, usefulness, and valence (positive vs. negative) of these beliefs, expectations, and other thoughts. Negatively skewed thinking patterns are strong determinants of health outcomes such as pain, function, and quality of life. One overly negative belief that influences illness behavior is called catastrophizing [16]. Catastrophizing is characterized by a tendency to exaggerate the threat value of aversive symptoms [12] such as pain, diarrhea, or urgency. Catastrophizing comprises 3 different cognitive elements: rumination (e.g. 'I can't stop thinking about how bad it would be'), magnification ('I worry that something serious may happen'), and helplessness ('There is nothing I can do to control it'). Catastrophizing has been most extensively studied in the context of chronic pain patients who tend to distort their evaluations of their own behavior and performance in an overly negative manner [17]. Sullivan and Neish [18] showed that catastrophizing scores predict pain and functional status (e.g. perceived disability, employment status). Drossman et al. [19] were one of the first research teams to extend the construct of catastrophizing to patients with FGIDs. They measured catastrophizing in patients with IBS, and found that it helped predict subsequent (12-month) health outcomes as measured by a composite health status of six variables (current pain, bed disability days, psychological distress, daily dysfunction, number of physician visits, number of surgeries and procedures) that was heavily weighted toward illness behaviors.

Another cognitive information processing variable that influences treatment seeking behavior are patients' worries. Worry is distinguished from pain catastrophizing on the basis of its uncontrollability, narrative quality, inherent future orientation, chronicity, and pervasiveness (i.e. problem topics are not specific to a single situation or stimuli). Whereas the focal problem underlying pain catastrophizing is by definition relatively well defined, worry is abstract, conceptual, and nonconcrete [20]. Unlike pain catastrophizing, worry functions as a way of avoiding perceived threat [21] that does not physically exist in the 'here and now' and for which there is no available behavioral response (e.g. escape). Worrying distracts from emotional distress and suppresses unpleasant somatic sensations in a manner that is negatively reinforcing and lends uncontrollability to the worry process. Difficulty controlling worry often results in prolonged bouts of worry that are difficult to 'turn off', which may cause significant distress and functional impairment. High levels of worry are associated with heightened focus on bodily symptoms, repeated checking for signs and symptoms related to health concerns, focus on the negative consequences of physical sensations, and frequent efforts to obtain reassurance from family members, friends, or health care professionals. FGID patients who worry that their GI symptoms (e.g. abdominal pain) signify an underlying physical disease (e.g. colon cancer) are more heavily represented among consulters than nonconsulters [22]. Gomborone et al. [23] compared illness attitudes (e.g. health worries) between patients with IBS and organic GI disease, and found that the IBS patients reported more health worries. The magnitude of health worry was not explained by the severity of either coexisting mental distress or somatic symptoms.

Levels of coexisting emotional distress can also influence the expression of illness behaviors [24]. Multiple studies of FGID patients recruited from tertiary care settings indicate that they are characterized by relatively high levels of anxiety, depression, or other forms of distress compared to nonconsulters [25]. Whitehead et al. [26] showed that treatment-seeking IBS patients had higher scores than normal subjects and nonconsulting individuals with IBS symptoms on multiple dimensions (anxiety, somatization, interpersonal sensitivity, etc.) of a psychiatric symptom checklist. Similar findings were reported by Drossman et al. [27]. Individuals with IBS symptoms who do not seek medical care for IBS symptoms generally have a normal psychological profile, although some studies show that their levels of psychological distress fall within intermediate levels (i.e. between normal and clinical ranges [28, 29]).

Psychiatric Comorbidity in IBD and Functional Gastrointestinal Disorders

Other researchers have approached the issue of psychiatric comorbidity by examining the proportion of FGID patients who meet diagnostic criteria for a formal mental disorder. Psychiatric comorbidity is relatively commonplace among FGID patients presenting at tertiary clinics. In studies [30] that have administered structured clinical interviews to establish the rate of psychiatric comorbidity among IBS patients per criteria as specified in the American Psychiatric Association's *Diagnostic and Statistical Manual of Mental Disorders* [31], approximately 60% of treatment-seeking IBS patients have a diagnosable psychiatric condition [32]. By comparison, approximately 25% of American adults suffer from a diagnosable mental disorder [33, 34].

The most frequent class of psychiatric diagnoses are the anxiety disorders. Within this class, the most prevalent anxiety disorders is generalized anxiety disorder (GAD) whose key defining feature is chronic feelings of intense (uncontrollable, excessive) worry concerning a range of different topics. For the individual with GAD, the target of worry is not limited to a single topic such as health concerns. The focus of worry may involve a generalized variety of daily life events due to (a) a sense that he/she is often unable to cope with those events or reactions to events; (b) fear of making mistakes or failing in any task of importance; and (c) concern with being negatively evaluated by oneself and by others. Intense worry is often accompanied by nervousness, physical tension, restlessness, and other symptoms of CNS arousal.

In addition to anxiety disorders, a significant proportion of IBS patients meet diagnostic criteria for a mood disorder. Between 12 and 28% meet criteria for major depressive disorder and 7% dysthymic disorder [35–37]. It is believed that negative mood states arising from psychiatric comorbidities may negatively bias interpretations of symptoms, which leads to increased symptom reporting and health care seeking [24]. Research that has attempted to identify the temporal relationship between onset of IBS and comorbid psychiatric diagnoses has found that mood disorders appear to precede the onset of IBS, whereas anxiety disorders typically follow IBS onset [38]. Other psychiatric comorbidities include somatoform disorders, a group of disorders that cause medically unexplained somatic symptoms [39].

Of course, even if up to 60% of treatment-seeking IBS patients have a psychiatric diagnosis, a substantial proportion (40%) do not have a formal mental illness. This means that psychiatric comorbidity alone is insufficient for fully understanding the contribution of psychological factors to FGIDs. This has prompted some researchers to shift the focus from distress emanating from comorbid psychiatric conditions to distress arising from GI-specific symptoms [40]. To this end, UCLA researchers have focused on the concept known as GI-specific anxiety. GI-specific anxiety refers to a fear of visceral sensations ('I often fear that I won't be able to have a normal bowel movement') and their consequences ('I get anxious when I go to a new restaurant') [41]. Situations that are likely to trigger GI symptom-specific anxiety include those involving food and eating such as restaurants and parties or locations where the availability of bathroom facilities is unknown. GI-specific anxiety is conceived as a marker of overresponsiveness to GI sensations which is believed to perpetuate IBS symptoms through alterations in autonomic and pain facilitation, as well as cognitive (e.g. attention, internal self-focus) mechanisms [41]. GI-specific anxiety may be associated with beliefs of poor symptom control and high illness impact and may, therefore, be a critical element in the severe decrements in quality of life found in IBS patients. GI-specific anxiety has been shown to be significantly associated with IBS severity and impact even after controlling for trait anxiety. GI symptom-specific anxiety is regarded as an especially important psychosocial variable underlying visceral pain sensitivity, hypervigilance, and maladaptive coping [40, 42]. It is unclear whether levels of visceral anxiety influence health care seeking.

Psychological Processes as Psychological Vulnerability Factors

A third pathway through which psychological factors influence IBS is by increasing the risk of developing IBS. In general, this line of research has focused on 3 types of psychosocial risk factors – negative learning experiences, personality traits, and life stress (trauma, stressors) [43]. One vulnerability factor may be a self-reported history of early-life adversity (e.g. physical and or sexual abuse).

Trauma History

A history of sexual abuse (as defined by nonconsensual sexual contact obtained through unwanted touching/fondling and physical contact with the sexual parts of the victim's or the offender's body through force or threat of harm or rape) and/or physical trauma (i.e. frequent beating, life threat) occurs in 20–60% of IBS patients seen in the US and Europe [44]. Drossman et al. [45] found that the frequency of a history of abuse among functional GI disorder patients was 30% greater than in women with an organic GI disease. Early-life adversity is believed to induce changes in the CNS, including altered function of the hypothalamic-pituitary-adrenal axis and the sympathetic nervous system, in genetically predisposed individuals [46, 47]. Additionally, trauma may cause epigenetic programming of glucocorticoid receptor expression that affects behavioral adaption to vulnerability to stress-related disorders. Information regarding abuse history is clinically important for a cohort of patients because it corresponds with refractory symptoms, greater healthcare utilization (e.g. more frequent visits to the doctor), and susceptibility to undergoing unneeded medical procedures [45, 48]. The high frequency of abuse is, however, not specific to IBS patients and is reported by patients with other persistent pain disorders such as fibromyalgia, headache or pelvic pain. In this respect, trauma is not a cause of IBS. At best, it can be understood as an early stressor that occurs with relatively high frequency and may predispose some individuals to adult-onset IBS and poorer outcomes.

Additional evidence supporting the role of a stress as a risk factor for IBS comes from studies [49] of patients who develop IBS after a bout of infectious gastroenteritis (i.e. postinfectious IBS or PI-IBS). Approximately 10% of patients with PI-IBS retrospectively attribute the onset of symptoms to an infectious illness [50]. While most patients rapidly recover from bacterial gastroenteritis, up to a third of patients experience persistent GI symptoms with a portion of those affected meeting diagnostic criteria for IBS [51]. Risk factors for developing PI-IBS include, in descending order of importance: duration of initial illness, toxicity of infecting bacterial strain, smoking, mucosal markers of inflammation, female gender, depression, hypochondriasis, and the occurrence of stressful life events (particularly interpersonal problems such as relationship breakup, loss) within 3 months of the infectious illness. Of 8 risk factors for onset of PI-IBS, 4 are psychosocial factors. These data are consistent with the work of Dunlop et al. [49] who found that the power of depression scores to independently predict PI-IBS rivaled rectal mucosal enterochromaffin cell count, suggesting that both biological and psychological factors are important in the development of PI-IBS. The underlying mechanisms whereby psychological factors increase the risk of PI-IBS are unclear, but one possibility is that they maintain low-grade inflammation.

Neuroticism

A number of researchers have focused attention on personality traits as risk factors for IBS. While there is no evidence of a unique IBS-prone personality, a proportion of individuals have a temperamental vulnerability that puts them at risk for developing IBS symptoms. The temperamental vulnerability that is most often linked with IBS is neuroticism (also referred to as negative emotionality or negative temperament). Neuroticism reflects a broad and pervasive personality dimension that helps explain individual differences in the propensity to experience negative emotions including sadness, fear, anxiety, anger, frustration, as well as associated characteristics including low self-esteem, worry and insecurity.

Neuroticism is associated with a tendency to experience negative affect in the face of minor stressors, to experience arousal quickly and difficulty returning to baseline following a period of evoked response. Physiologically, elevated neuroticism is associated with increased autonomic and neural responses to negative stimuli [52–54].

Cognitively, persons with high scores on neuroticism scales tend to have an internal self-focus (i.e. somatically focused) and a propensity to interpret noxious bodily sensations in a negative manner. On self-report measure, high neuroticism individuals report more bothersome symptoms, interpret their symptoms as more severe and express more general emotional distress than low neuroticism individuals. It is not surprising then that neuroticism has emerged as a psychological risk factor for a variety of emotional disorders and physical conditions [55].

In the case of FGIDs, a number of studies have documented the link between neuroticism and IBS [29, 56]. High scores on neuroticism scales characterize individuals with IBS symptoms [57], and neuroticism is regarded as a risk factor for chronic unexplained pain in IBS. Neuroticism may influence IBS experience by lowering the sensitivity threshold at which noxious symptoms (e.g. pain) are perceived as threatening, intolerable, and requiring medical intervention. Consistent with this hypothesis are findings from a study [58] comparing personality style of normal individuals, lactose malabsorbers (LMAs), and individuals with IBS in the general community who do not seek medical attention, versus LMAs and individuals with IBS who do seek healthcare. Higher rates of neuroticism characterized both LMAs and patients with IBS who sought medical assistance. The precise mechanisms underlying the effects of neuroticism on treatment seeking and other illness behaviors of IBS patients are not well established. Candidate explanations include increased awareness of somatic sensations, catastrophic appraisal of benign sensations as dangerous, and corresponding lower threshold for seeking medical care. Other researchers have argued that neuroticism confers a proneness to distress that can aggravate somatic sensations [59].

Observational Learning

Working from a social learning theory (SLT) perspective [60], Whitehead et al. [61] emphasize negative learning experiences in the etiology of FGIDs. SLT is the prevailing theoretical framework used in health behavior and health promotion research. In SLT, human behavior is explained in terms of a three-way, dynamic, reciprocal theory in which individual (e.g. biology, emotions, cognitions) factors, environmental influences, and behavior interact continually. A basic premise of SLT is that people learn not only through their own experiences but also by observing the actions of others (i.e. observational learning, modeling) and the results of those actions (consequences). The family environment is a fertile context in which learning occurs. Whitehead et al. [62] contend that complaints of IBS symptoms are partly acquired by children who learn through direct experience and by observing how others (e.g. parents) respond to IBS. In support of the general principle of familial transmission are results of a large telephone survey that found that individuals who reported IBS-like symptoms were likely to recall that their parents both responded to GI symptoms such as stomach aches with the provision of positive reinforcement (e.g. gifts, toys) and demonstrated illness behaviors (school absences, physician visits) that can negatively reinforce symptoms. Similarly, Levy et al. [63] found that children of IBS parents sought medical care for GI and non-GI complaints more than matched controls. These data are consistent with the notion that experience of IBS is to some extent shaped by negative learning experiences formed in the family environment [64].

Psychological Treatments as Evidence-Based Treatments

The fourth pathway linking psychological factors to IBS is through the application of psychological techniques to relieve IBS symptoms and related distress. In essence, psychological treatments are specifically designed to alter psychological processes thought to underlie or significantly contribute to pain, distress, and disability or normalize gut function. The most well-studied psychological treatment is a specific therapy called cognitive behavior therapy or CBT. The cognitive part of CBT helps people change specific thinking patterns that heighten physiological and psychological arousal, while the behavioral part helps people change the way they react to situational triggers. CBT techniques (e.g. cognitive restructuring, relaxation techniques) have been administered either singularly or in combination with other interventions and have been featured in over 30 randomized clinical trials since 1985. CBT generally yields broad improvements in GI symptoms (pain, bowel dysfunction) and quality of life. Research summarized in a recent systematic review suggests that psychological treatments as a whole are at least moderately effective in reducing IBS symptoms [65, 66]. Whether treatment gains following a regimen of CBT are enduring in the longer term is unclear. Although there were not enough data to establish the relative superiority of any one type of psychological treatment, most trials featured CBT. A recent study using CBT to treat severely affected IBS patients found that the great majority of patients reported significant reduction in the severity of IBS symptoms and reported adequate relief from IBS symptoms [67]. The therapeutic value of CBT was echoed in a recently published *New England Journal of Medicine* [68] narrative review that identified CBT as one of the few empirically validated treatments for IBS. Other evidence-based psychological treatments include hypnosis and interpersonal psychotherapy [69].

Acknowledgements

This study was supported in part by a research grant from the National Institutes of Health, NIDDK (DK77738).

References

1 Chang L: Review article: epidemiology and quality of life in functional gastrointestinal disorders. Aliment Pharmacol Ther 2004;20(suppl 7):31–39.

2 Drossman DA, Sandler RS, McKee DC, et al: Bowel patterns among subjects not seeking health care. Use of a questionnaire to identify a population with bowel dysfunction. Gastroenterology 1982;83:529–534.

3 Thompson WG, Heaton KW: Functional bowel disorders in apparently healthy people. Gastroenterology 1980;79:283–288.

4 Drossman DA: Presidential address: gastrointestinal illness and the biopsychosocial model. Psychosom Med 1997;60:258–267.

5 Van Oudenhove L, Aziz Q: The role of psychosocial factors and psychiatric disorders in functional dyspepsia. Nat Rev Gastroenterol Hepatol 2013;10:158–167.

6 Chang L: The role of stress on physiologic responses and clinical symptoms in irritable bowel syndrome. Gastroenterology 2011;140:761–765 e5.

7 Almy TP, Kern F, Tulin M: Alterations in colonic function in man under stress. II. Experimental production of sigmoid spasm in healthy persons. Gastroenterology 1949;12:425–436.

8 Welgan P, Meshkinpour H, Beeler M: Effect of anger on colon motor and myoelectric activity in irritable bowel syndrome. Gastroenterology 1988;94:1150–1156.

9 Welgan P, Meshkinpour H, Hoehler F: The effect of stress on colon motor and electrical activity in irritable bowel syndrome. Psychosom Med 1985;47:139–149.

10 Dickhaus B, Mayer EA, Firooz N, et al: Irritable bowel syndrome patients show enhanced modulation of visceral perception by auditory stress. Am J Gastroenterol 2003;98:135–143.

11 Murray CDR, Flynn J, Ratcliffe L, et al: Effect of acute physical and psychological stress on gut autonomic innervation in irritable bowel syndrome. Gastroenterology 2004;127:1695–1703.

12 Bennet EJ, Tennant CC, Piesse C, et al: Level of chronic life stress predicts clinical outcome in irritable bowel syndrome. Gut 1998;43:256–261.

13 Creed F, Craig T, Farmer R: Functional abdominal pain, psychiatric illness, and life events. Gut 1988;29:235–242.

14 Pilowsky I: The diagnosis of abnormal illness behaviour. Aust N Z J Psychiatry 1971;5:136–138.

15 Levy RL, Whitehead WE, Von Korff MR, et al: Intergenerational transmission of gastrointestinal illness behavior. Am J Gastroenterol 2000;95:451–456.

16 Turner JA, Aaron LA: Pain-related catastrophizing: what is it? Clin J Pain 2001;17:65–71.

17 Lefebvre MF: Cognitive distortion and cognitive errors in depressed psychiatric and low back pain patients. J Consult Clin Psychol 1981;49:517–525.

18 Sullivan M, Neish NR: Catastrophizing, anxiety and pain during dental hygiene treatment. Community Dent Oral Epidemiol 1998;26:344–349.

19 Drossman DA, Li Z, Leserman J, et al: Effects of coping on health outcome among female patients with gastrointestinal disorders. Psychosom Med 2000;62:309–317.

20 Kindt M, Brosschot JF, Boiten F: High-Level cognition in phobics: abstract anticipatory memory is associated with the attenuation of physiological reactivity to threat. J Anxiety Disord 1999;13:473–489.

21 Borkovec TD, Hu S: The effect of worry on cardiovascular response to phobic imagery. Behav Res Ther 1990;28:69–73.

22 Creed FH, Levy RL, Bradley LA, et al (eds): Psychosocial Aspects of Functional Gastrointestinal Disorders. McLean, Degnon Associates, 2006.

23 Gomborone J, Dewsnap P, Libby G, et al: Abnormal illness attitudes in patients with irritable bowel syndrome. J Psychosom Res 1995;39:227–230.

24 Cohen S, Rodriguez M: Pathways linking affective disturbances and physical disorders. Health Psychol 1995;14:374–380.

25 Koloski NA, Talley NJ, Boyce PM: Epidemiology and health care seeking in the functional GI disorders: a population-based study. Am J Gastroenterol 2002;97:2290–2299.

26 Whitehead WE, Bosmajian L, Zonderman AB, et al: Symptoms of psychologic distress associated with irritable bowel syndrome. Comparison of community and medical clinic samples. Gastroenterology 1988;95:709–714.

27 Drossman DA, McKee DC, Sandler RS, et al: Psychosocial factors in the irritable bowel syndrome. A multivariate study of patients and nonpatients with irritable bowel syndrome. Gastroenterology 1988;95:701–708.

28 Mertz H: Role of the brain and sensory pathways in gastrointestinal sensory disorders in humans. Gut 2002;51(suppl 1):i29–i33.

29 Talley NJ, Boyce PM, Jones M: Is the association between irritable bowel syndrome and abuse explained by neuroticism? A population based study. Gut 1998;42:47–53.

30 Blanchard EB: Irritable Bowel Syndrome: Psychosocial Assessment and Treatment. Washington, American Psychiatric Association, 2000.

31 American Psychiatric Association: Diagnostic and Statistical Manual of Mental Disorders, ed 4. Washington, American Psychiatric Association, 1994.
32 Blanchard EB, Scharff L: Psychosocial aspects of assessment and treatment of irritable bowel syndrome in adults and recurrent abdominal pain in children. J Consult Clin Psychol 2002;70:725–738.
33 Alegria M, Jackson JS, Kessler RS, et al: National Comorbidity Survey Replication (NCS-R) 2001–2003. Ann Arbor, Inter-University Consortium for Political and Social Research, 2003.
34 Kessler RC, Berglund P, Chiu WT, et al: The US National Comorbidity Survey Replication (NCS-R): design and field procedures. Int J Methods Psychiatr Res 2004;13:69–92.
35 Lydiard RB, Fossey MD, Marsh W, et al: Prevalence of psychiatric disorders in patients with irritable bowel syndrome. Psychosomatics 1993;34:229–234.
36 Canavan JB, Bennett K, Feely J, et al: Significant psychological morbidity occurs in irritable bowel syndrome: a case-control study using a pharmacy reimbursement database. Aliment Pharmacol Ther 2009;29:440–449.
37 Ballenger JC, Davidson JR, Lecrubier Y, et al: Consensus statement on depression, anxiety, and functional gastrointestinal disorders. J Clin Psychiatry 2001;62(suppl 8):48–51.
38 Sykes MA, Blanchard EB, Lackner J, et al: Psychopathology in irritable bowel syndrome: support for a psychophysiological model. J Behav Med 2003;26:361–372.
39 Miller AR, North CS, Clouse RE, et al: The association of irritable bowel syndrome and somatization disorder. Ann Clin Psychiatry 2001;13:25–30.
40 Labus JS, Mayer EA, Chang L, et al: The central role of gastrointestinal-specific anxiety in irritable bowel syndrome: further validation of the visceral sensitivity index. Psychosom Med 2007;69:89–98.
41 Labus JS, Mayer EA, Chang L, et al: The central role of gastrointestinal-specific anxiety in irritable bowel syndrome: further validation of the Visceral Sensitivity Index. Psychosom Med 2007;69:89–98.
42 Labus JS, Bolus R, Chang L, et al: The Visceral Sensitivity Index: development and validation of a gastrointestinal symptom-specific anxiety scale. Aliment Pharmacol Ther 2004;20:89–97.
43 Drossman DA: Irritable bowel syndrome. Gastroenterologist 1994;2:315–326.
44 Drossman DA: Abuse, trauma, and GI illness: is there a link? Am J Gastroenterol 2011;106:14–25.
45 Drossman DA, Leserman J, Nachman G, et al: Sexual and physical abuse in women with functional or organic gastrointestinal disorders. Ann Intern Med 1990;113:828–833.
46 Chang L, Sundaresh S, Elliott J, et al: Dysregulation of the hypothalamic-pituitary-adrenal (HPA) axis in irritable bowel syndrome. Neurogastroenterol Motil 2009;21:149–159.
47 Videlock EJ, Adeyemo M, Licudine A, et al: Childhood trauma is associated with hypothalamic-pituitary-adrenal axis responsiveness in irritable bowel syndrome. Gastroenterology 2009;137:1954–1962.
48 Drossman DA, Talley N, Leserman J, et al: Sexual and physical abuse and gastrointestinal illness: review and recommendations. Ann Intern Med 1995;123:782–789.
49 Dunlop SP, Jenkins D, Neal KR, et al: Relative importance of enterochromaffin cell hyperplasia, anxiety, and depression in postinfectious IBS. Gastroenterology 2003;125:1651–1659.
50 Collins SM, Vallance B, Barbara G, et al: Putative inflammatory and immunological mechanisms in functional bowel disorders. Baillieres Best Pract Res Clin Gastroenterol 1999;13:429–436.
51 Spiller R, Garsed K: Infection, inflammation, and the irritable bowel syndrome. Dig Liver Dis 2009;41:844–849.
52 Coen SJ, Kano M, Farmer AD, et al: Neuroticism influences brain activity during the experience of visceral pain. Gastroenterology 2011;141:909–917 e1.
53 Canli T: Functional brain mapping of extraversion and neuroticism: learning from individual differences in emotion processing. J Pers 2004;72:1105–1132.
54 Norris CJ, Larsen JT, Cacioppo JT: Neuroticism is associated with larger and more prolonged electrodermal responses to emotionally evocative pictures. Psychophysiology 2007;44:823–826.
55 Charles ST, Gatz M, Kato K, et al: Physical health 25 years later: the predictive ability of neuroticism. Health Psychol 2008;27:369–378.
56 Talley NJ, Boyce PM, Jones M: Predictors of health care seeking for irritable bowel syndrome: a population based study. Gut 1997;41:394–398.
57 Hazlett-Stevens H, Craske MG, Mayer EA, et al: Prevalence of irritable bowel syndrome among university students: the roles of worry, neuroticism, anxiety sensitivity and visceral anxiety. J Psychosom Res 2003;55:501–505.
58 Enck P, Holtkotter B, Whitehead W, et al: Clinical symptoms, psychopathology and intestinal motility in patients with 'irritable bowel' (in German). Z Gastroenterol 1989;27:357–361.
59 Wade JB, Price DD: Nonpathological factors in chronic pain: implications for assessment and treatment; in Gatchel RJ, Weisberg JN (eds): Personality Characteristics of Patients with Pain. Washington, American Psychological Association, 2000.
60 Bandura A: Self-efficacy: toward a unifying theory of behavioral change. Psychol Rev 1977;84:191–215.

61 Whitehead WE, Bosmajian L, Zonderman AB, et al: Symptoms of psychologic distress associated with irritable bowel syndrome: comparison of community and medical clinical samples. Gastroenterology 1988;95:709–714.

62 Whitehead WE, Winget C, Fedoravicius AS, et al: Learned illness behavior in patients with irritable bowel syndrome and peptic ulcer. Dig Dis Sci 1982; 27:202–208.

63 Levy RL, Whitehead WE, Walker LS, et al: Increased somatic complaints and health-care utilization in children: effects of parent IBS status and parent response to gastrointestinal symptoms. Am J Gastroenterol 2004;99:2442–2451.

64 Chitkara DK, van Tilburg MAL, Blois-Martin N, et al: Early life risk factors that contribute to irritable bowel syndrome in adults: a systematic review. Am J Gastroenterol 2008;103:765–774.

65 Ford AC, Vandvik PO: Irritable bowel syndrome. Clin Evid (Online) 2012;2012:pii 0410.

66 Lackner JM, Morley S, Dowzer C, et al: Psychological treatments for irritable bowel syndrome: a systematic review and meta-analysis. J Consult Clin Psychol 2004;72:1100–1113.

67 Lackner JM, Jaccard J, Krasner SS, et al: Self-administered cognitive behavior therapy for moderate to severe irritable bowel syndrome: clinical efficacy, tolerability, feasibility. Clin Gastroenterol Hepatol 2008;6:899–906.

68 Mayer EA: Clinical practice. Irritable bowel syndrome. N Engl J Med 2008;358:1692–1699.

69 Naliboff B, Lackner JM, Mayer E: Psychosocial factors in the care of patients with functional gastrointestinal disorders; in Yamada T (ed): Principles of Clinical Gastroenterology. New York, John Wiley & Sons, 2008, pp 20–37.

Jeffrey M. Lackner, Psy.D.
Behavioral Medicine Clinic, Department of Medicine, UB School of Medicine, SUNY
ECMC, 462 Grider Street
Buffalo, NY 14215 (USA)
E-Mail lackner@buffalo.edu

Quigley EMM, Hongo M, Fukudo S (eds): Functional and GI Motility Disorders.
Front Gastrointest Res. Basel, Karger, 2014, vol 33, pp 117–129 (DOI: 10.1159/000356788)

The Pharmacology of the Gut-Brain Axis: Prospects for Future Therapeutic Progress?

Scott Gabbard · Brian E. Lacy

Division of Gastroenterology and Hepatology, Dartmouth-Hitchcock Medical Center, Lebanon, N.H., USA

Abstract

The brain-gut axis is the bidirectional communication system that includes the central nervous system, the enteric nervous system, the wall and lumen of the gastrointestinal (GI) tract, and the hypothalamo-pituitary-adrenal axis. This active bidirectional highway links emotional and cognitive centers in the brain with the GI tract. In health, the brain-gut axis is important for regulating appetite, food intake, gut immune function, and the coordination of GI tract function with the emotional state of the organism. In a variety of disease states, the normal physiology of the brain-gut axis may be disturbed, and this can lead to changes in gut motility, secretion and immune function. Disruption of normal brain-gut axis physiology plays a role in the generation of many GI symptoms, including abdominal pain, bloating, diarrhea and constipation. These symptoms are commonly found in patients classified as having functional GI disorders (FGIDs). FGIDs are characterized by recurrent symptoms in GI tract that cannot be explained by currently available endoscopic, radiologic, or biochemical tests. FGIDs are highly prevalent; conservative estimates are that at least 40% of the population has symptoms of at least one FGID. To date, 28 separate FGIDs have been defined and characterized in adults, and this includes the two most clinically relevant FGIDs, irritable bowel syndrome and functional dyspepsia. For years, treatment for most FGIDs focused simply on medications that targeted the GI tract. Recognition of the key role that the brain-gut axis plays in symptom generation in FGID patients has opened up new avenues for therapeutic intervention. This review will briefly summarize new treatment options that focus on the brain-gut axis, with an emphasis on FGIDs.

Non-Gastroesophageal Reflux Disease Esophageal Disorders

Functional chest pain (FCP) of presumed esophageal origin is a heterogeneous disorder thought to be secondary to multiple factors including reflux, esophageal spasm, and visceral hypersensitivity. The overall prevalence of FCP has been estimated to be 13–23% [1, 2]. FCP has been demonstrated to reduce quality of life (QOL) to levels similar to those of patients with a cardiac etiology for their pain [3]; total healthcare costs for FCP have been estimated to exceed USD 300 million annually [4]. Current treatment options for FCP not due to gastroesophageal reflux disease (GERD) include smooth muscle relaxants and pain modulators; however, there are limited data demonstrating minimal efficacy for their use in FCP [5]. Current studies are focused on modulation of central and peripheral nocioceptive pathways through pharmacologic and homeopathic mechanisms.

TRPV1 Antagonists

Transient receptor potential vanilloid 1 (TRPV1) has been postulated to be involved in nocioception of acid in the esophagus [6]; antagonism of TRPV1 has been an attractive target for treatment of FCP. However, a recent placebo-controlled, double-blinded, crossover phase 2 trial of 14 patients with nonerosive reflux disease (NERD) and partial response to proton pump inhibitor (PPI) with the TRPV1 antagonist AZD1386 showed no change in the pain threshold for heat, distension, or electrical current compared to placebo [7]. Development of this medication has been halted, and it remains to be seen if other TRPV1 antagonists will be developed.

ONO-8539

Prostaglandin E_2 (PGE2) EP1 has previously been shown to contribute to esophageal pain hypersensitivity [8, 9]. ONO-8539 is a PGE2 EP1 receptor antagonist currently in phase I study for hypersensitivity in NERD (ClinicalTrials.gov NCT01707901). ONO-8539 was previously studied for overactive bladder; unfortunately, it had little impact on symptom relief in a phase III study.

Cannabis

Cannabis modulates visceral pain transmission through the suppression of nociceptive processing via activation of cannabinoid receptors CB1 and CB2. CB1 may also decrease transient lower esophageal sphincter relaxations (TLESRs) through modulation of vagal pathways [10]. Dronabinol is currently being studied in a placebo-controlled phase 4 trial in 40 patients with noncardiac, nonreflux chest pain (ClinicalTrials.gov NCT01598207).

Hypnotherapy

Hypnotherapy administered weekly by a therapist has previously been demonstrated to decrease both global and chest pain [11]. It is postulated that hypnotherapy may normalize visceral sensation and decrease contractile activity in the gut. Currently, there is a trial of home administered hypnotherapy (HHT) comparing HHT to a home educational program regarding functional gastrointestinal disorders (FGIDs; ClinicalTrials.gov NCT01284179).

Gastroesophageal Reflux Disease

According to the Montreal Classification, GERD is defined as a condition that develops when the reflux of stomach contents causes troublesome symptoms and/or complications [12]. One of the most common gastrointestinal (GI) disorders, GERD has an estimated prevalence of 10–28% [13, 14]. GERD has been shown to decrease QOL compared to those without [15]; importantly, those who respond to PPI have increased QOL compared with nonresponders [16]. Current medical therapy of GERD centers on decreasing gastric acid secretion via PPIs or histamine type 2 receptor antagonists. Over the past decade, various medications designed to inhibit TLESRs have been studied; to date, none has demonstrated benefit in a phase III trial.

TLESR Inhibitors

Arbaclofen placarbil, thought to inhibit TLESR through GABA9B activation, failed to demonstrate a significant difference in weekly heartburn when compared to placebo over 4 weeks of treatment [17]. ADX10059, a metabotropic glutamate receptor 5 (mGluR5) negative allosteric modulator, had been shown in a phase IIB study to reduce reflux events and improve reflux symptoms [18]; however, development of the drug was halted due to hepatotoxicity in longer-term studies.

A large multicenter randomized, placebo-controlled trial is currently underway comparing Nissen fundoplication to a combination of baclofen and desipramine in patients with persistent GERD symptoms despite PPI. Baclofen has previously been demonstrated to decrease TLESRs [19]; however, its use is somewhat limited by sedation. The study has aimed to recruit nearly 400 patients at 15 VA hospitals across the US (ClinicalTrials.gov NCT01265550).

SSP-002358

The 5-HT_4 agonist tegaserod was previously found to decrease postprandial acid exposure in the distal esophagus. This effect was postulated to be due to a decrease in gastric emptying time as well as a decrease in TLESRs [20]. While tegaserod is not available in North America, another 5-HT_4 agonist, SSP-002358, is currently being studied in combination with PPI in a phase IIb study for patients with persistent regurgitation despite PPI therapy (ClinicalTrials.gov NCT01472939).

Functional Dyspepsia

Functional dyspepsia (FD) is a highly prevalent disorder that reduces patients' QOL [for a full review, see the chapter by Tack, pp. 38–44]. Despite its worldwide prevalence of approximately 10%, and its significant impact on patients and the global health care system, no medication is currently approved in the US, Canada, or the European Union for the treatment of FD. However, recent clinical trials have provided new information on potential therapeutic options for FD.

Acotiamide

Acotiamide enhances acetylcholine release from enteric neurons through muscarinic receptor antagonism and acetycholinesterase inhibition [21] and has been demonstrated in Japan to increase both the gastric accommodation reflex as well as accelerate gastric emptying in patients who fit Rome II criteria for FD [22]. In a phase III, randomized, placebo-controlled trial in patients who met Rome III criteria for FD-PDS, acotiamide at a dose of 100 mg t.i.d. for 4 weeks significantly decreased overall symptoms and meal-related symptoms as well as increased QOL scores compared with placebo [23]. Additionally, there was no rebound or relapse of symptoms when the medication was stopped after 4 weeks. In both studies, acotiamide was well tolerated and had a similar rate of adverse events compared to placebo.

IW-9179

Guanylate cyclase type C (GC-G) agonists have been demonstrated to reduce visceral pain in rodent models via modulation of afferent nerve activity through cGMP [24, 25]. IW-9179, a second generation GC-G, is currently being evaluated in a phase IIa study in FD patients (ClinicalTrials.gov NCT01712412).

Gastroparesis

The etiology, pathophysiology, and impact of gastroparesis (GP) are discussed in full in the chapter by Parkman [pp. 25–37]. Two new agents that modulate different aspects of the brain-gut axis are currently under investigation and are described below.

TZP-102

Ghrelin is produced in response to eating and enhances gastric motility in both animals and humans [26–28]. TZP-102 is an oral macrocyclic compound that acts as a potent ghrelin agonist. A recent, 28-day, double-blind, multicenter study in 92 patients with diabetic GP evaluated the efficacy of 3 doses of TZP-102 (10, 20, and 40 mg) compared to placebo for both symptoms and gastric emptying using a 13C breath test [29]. The authors reported that the once-daily medication was well tolerated and that all doses improved symptoms, using the Gastroparesis Cardinal Symptom Index, compared to placebo. Gastric emptying was not changed compared to baseline at any dose. Larger studies will be required to confirm these preliminary results and to determine whether this drug is efficacious only in patients with diabetic GP, or in all categories of GP.

RM-131

RM-131 is a novel small synthetic pentapeptide that acts as a ghrelin receptor agonist. In a rat model of postoperative ileus, RM-131 was more effective than human ghrelin at reversing gastric ileus, and in healthy primates, RM-131 increased gastric emptying. Data in humans are quite limited [30]. A phase II, randomized, double-blind, placebo-controlled study is currently underway to assess the safety and efficacy of RM-131 in patients with diabetic GP (ClinicalTrials.gov NCT01571297).

Irritable Bowel Syndrome

Irritable bowel syndrome (IBS) is a highly prevalent functional bowel disorder routinely encountered by all health care providers. Although not life threatening, this chronic disorder reduces patients' QOL and imposes a significant economic burden on the health care system. IBS should be confidently diagnosed in the clinic at the time of the first office visit using the Rome III criteria in conjunction with a careful history and physical examination. Treatment options for IBS have increased in number in the past decade; many of these modulate brain-gut axis function.

Tricyclic Antidepressants

Tricyclic antidepressants (TCAs) have been used to treat functional bowel disorders for over three decades. There are several reasons why TCAs might influence the brain-gut axis and improve functional GI symptoms. One, TCAs have a central analgesic effect. Two, TCAs may improve sleep, and this is important as disordered sleep can alter sensory thresholds. Three, TCAs can positively alter mood, and psychological disorders of anxiety, depression, and somatization are common in patients with FGIDs. Four, TCAs have peripheral analgesic effects. Finally, TCAs may promote smooth muscle relaxation in some patients (e.g. fundic relaxation in patients with FD). In the central nervous system (CNS), these drugs inhibit the reuptake of serotonin (5-HT) and norepinephrine. However, these agents also have effects on multiple other neurotransmitter pathways. The secondary amine TCAs (e.g. nortriptyline and desipramine) are generally better tolerated than their parent tertiary amine compounds (e.g. amitriptyline), given a lower propensity for anticholinergic, antihistamine, and α-adrenergic side effects. Only 7 studies have been conducted to date, and many of these were of limited duration and included only a small number of patients [31, 32]. In addition, side effects frequently develop as the dose is increased, and these side effects include dry mouth, dry eyes, sedation, urinary retention, and visual changes. Concerns over potential cardiac arrhythmias and the risk of overdose, accidental or intentional, have also been raised. The best data supporting the use of TCAs in the treatment of IBS are from a large placebo-controlled study evaluating desipramine for the treatment of functional bowel disorders in women. Although the intention-to-treat analysis did not show a statistically significant benefit compared to placebo (secondary to the dropout rate due to side effects), the per protocol analysis did show significant benefits compared to placebo [33]. This highlights the fact that if a patient can tolerate some of the side effects of a TCA, then he or she is more likely to note an improvement in chronic abdominal pain compared to a patient treated with placebo.

Selective Serotonin Reuptake Inhibitors and Serotonin-Norepinephrine Reuptake Inhibitors

Data on the use of selective serotonin reuptake inhibitors (SSRIs) and serotonin-norepinephrine reuptake inhibitors (SNRIs) in the treatment of IBS are even more limited than available data on the use of TCAs. Only 6 studies have been conducted to date, 2 each involving fluoxetine, paroxetine and citalopram [34–39]. Most patients noted an improvement in overall well-being, although none of the studies showed any benefit with regard to bowel habits, and abdominal pain was generally not improved. The paroxetine study provided some of the first evidence supporting the use of SSRIs in treating functional bowel disorders. One citalopram trial employed a controlled, crossover design and demonstrated a significant improvement in abdominal pain, bloating, and general well-being independent of psychological improvement [38]. It is felt that SSRIs primarily mediate pain centrally, but they may also have effects on the enteric nervous system (ENS). SSRIs are generally prescribed at dosages standard for treating mental health disorders. Only one trial performed a head-to-head comparison between a TCA (imipramine 50 mg) and an SSRI (citalopram 40 mg); neither drug demonstrated significant improvements in global IBS symptoms over placebo [39]. In other studies, both TCAs and SSRIs have been shown to improve IBS symptoms independently of depression and anxiety measures [40, 41]. Duloxetine, an SNRI, is used to treat depression and chronic pain syndromes. Fifteen IBS patients (Rome III criteria; all subtypes) were treated with duloxetine (30 mg for 1 week and then 60 mg for 11 weeks) in an open-label trial [42]. Eight patients completed the study; 7 withdrew due to adverse events (nausea, insomnia, constipation). The authors reported that duloxetine improved abdominal pain, severity of illness and loose stools in those who completed the study.

Gabapentin and Pregabalin

Gabapentin, an antiepileptic agent, amplifies GABA transmission and improves neuropathic pain by blocking $\alpha_2\delta$ voltage-dependent calcium channels and reducing the effects of central neurotransmitters such as glutamate, substance P, noradrenaline, and calcitonin gene-related peptide [43]. Pregabalin, structurally related to gabapentin, is approved for the management of certain pain disorders and as an adjunct for partial-onset seizures and generalized anxiety. Studies suggest these drugs impact the central processing of pain, and may alter autonomic function. In a short prospective study of 40 IBS-D patients (Rome II criteria), gabapentin (300 mg/day for 3 days and then 600 mg/day for 2 days) reduced rectal sensory thresholds and improved rectal compliance [44]. In another small study of IBS patients (n = 26) randomized to increasing doses of pregabalin (50–200 mg t.i.d. over 3 weeks) or placebo, patients treated with pregabalin noted improvements in rectal compliance and an increase in sensory thresholds for pain [45].

Dextofisopam

Dextofisopam is an atypical benzodiazepine that binds to the 2,3 benzodiazepine receptor in the CNS. It appears to reduce visceral pain and slow GI transit in animal models. A recent pilot study evaluated the safety and efficacy of dextofisopam in the treatment of men and women with IBS-M and IBS-D (n = 140; 73% female). Patients treated with dextofisopam (200 mg b.i.d.) noted adequate relief of global

IBS symptoms at the end of month 1 ($p = 0.002$), but not at months 2 or 3, when compared to placebo [46]. Stool frequency also improved during the first month of therapy in women, but not men, treated with this novel agent. Bloating was not improved in either men or women. Large prospective trials are needed to confirm these preliminary findings, and it is possible that this medication will find a role for the treatment of IBS-M symptoms, especially if used for short periods of time or on a p.r.n. basis.

Asimadoline

Asimadoline is a peripheral κ-opioid agonist. It is thought to have both analgesic and antidiarrheal effects, which makes it a potentially attractive therapeutic agent for patients with IBS-D. In a small, crossover trial in IBS patients, a single dose of asimadoline (0.5 mg) improved pain caused by colonic distention [47]. In a phase IIb randomized, placebo-controlled, dose-ranging (0.15, 0.5, 1 mg) study in men and women with all IBS subtypes, twice-daily asimadoline was no better than placebo using an intent-to-treat analysis [48]. However, when the data were analyzed further, IBS-D patients with at least moderate pain at baseline had a significant improvement in abdominal pain, stool frequency urgency and bloating, when compared to baseline. A large, prospective, phase III multicenter trial is needed to confirm these encouraging results in IBS patients with diarrhea predominance.

MuDelta

This novel agent is a locally acting mu opioid receptor agonist and delta opioid receptor antagonist in development for the treatment of IBS with diarrhea. Theoretically, the combination agent should improve abdominal pain and also symptoms of diarrhea by slowing GI transit, without causing significant constipation. In a phase II prospective, double-blind, placebo-controlled, dose-ranging study, 807 patients (Rome III criteria) were randomized to receive 1 of 4 doses of MuDelta (5, 25, 100, or 200 mg) or placebo twice daily. The primary end point of this 12-week study was an improvement in stool consistency and abdominal pain at week 4. Although all data are not yet available in peer-reviewed form, the sponsors reported that IBS-D patients (both men and women) who received either the 100 mg b.i.d. dose (28 vs. 13.9%) or the 200 mg b.i.d. dose (28.7 vs. 13.9%) were more likely than those receiving placebo to meet the primary end point ($p = 0.002$ for both doses). Two large multicenter phase III trials potentially involving more than 2,000 patients are currently in progress and should be completed by the end of 2013.

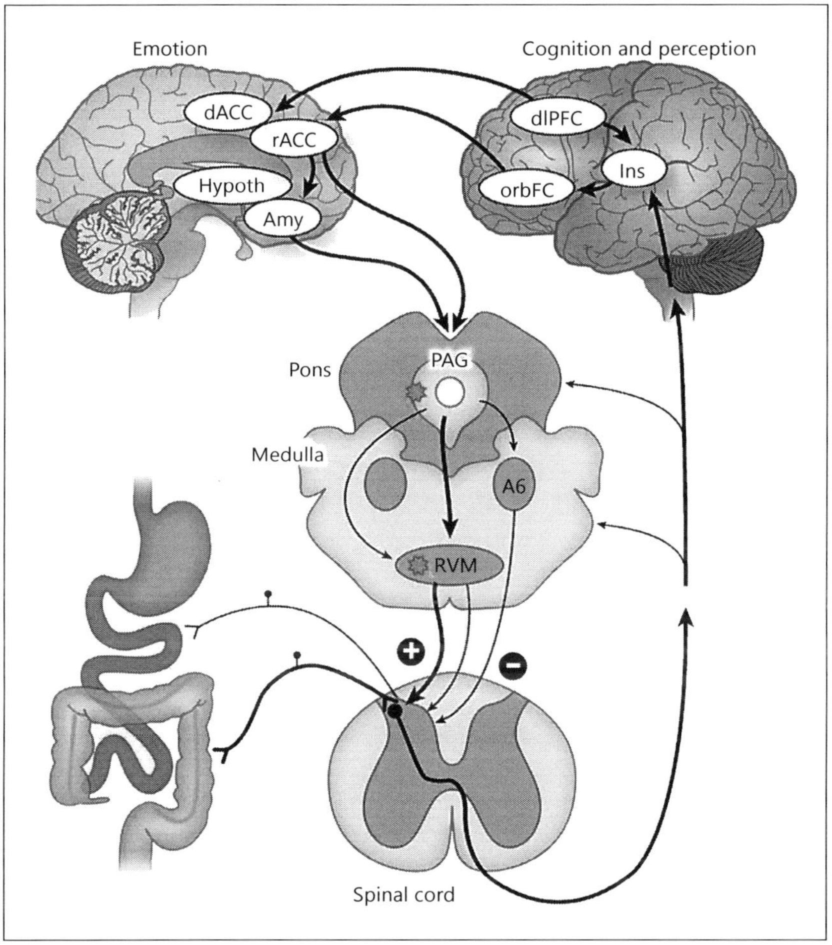

Fig. 1. Cortical modulation of homeostatic afferent input to the CNS. Prefrontal regions modulate activity in limbic and paralimbic regions, subregions of the anterior cingulate cortex, and hypothalamus, which in turn regulate the activity of descending inhibitory and facilitatory descending pathways through the periaqueductal gray and pontomedullary nuclei. Activity in these corticolimbic pontine networks mediates the effect of cognitions and emotions on the perception of homeostatic feelings, including visceral pain and discomfort. dlPFC = Dorsolateral PFC; orbFC = orbitofrontal cortex; PAG = periaqueductal gray; RVM = rostroventral medulla; A6 = locus coeruleus; Ins = insula; Hypoth = hypothalamus; Amy = amygdala; ACC = anterior cingulate cortex. Adapted from Mayer and Tillisch [58], with permission.

Tryptophan Hydroxylase Inhibitors – LX-1031

5-HT is known to play a critical role in GI tract sensation and motility, and previous studies have found that some IBS-D patients may have high circulating levels of serotonin [49]. LX-1031 directly inhibits 5-HT synthesis in the GI tract and thus has the potential to improve symptoms in patients with nonconstipation

IBS. In a phase II dose-ranging trial, LX-1031 (1,000 mg q.i.d. for 4 weeks) was superior to placebo at improving stool consistency in nonconstipation IBS patients [50]. Larger trials using FDA-mandated end points will be required to confirm these results.

Neurokinin Receptors

Substance P and neurokinin receptors play an important role in visceral pain and stress in both animals and humans. Neurokinin-1 receptors (NK1R) are located throughout the brain-gut axis (CNS, ENS, spinal pathways) and appear to be involved in brain regions critical to autonomic function and emotion [51]. A recent pilot study by Tillisch et al. [51] demonstrated that an NK1R antagonist decreased anxiety and pain in women with IBS, possibly through downregulation of central neural circuits involved in emotion and pain. These promising results warrant further investigation.

ATI-7505 (Naronapride)

Naronapride is an orally active 5-HT_4 receptor partial agonist that does not appear to have any significant activity on cardiac repolarization [52]. Naronapride increases gastric and colonic motility in healthy volunteers and improves stool frequency in patients with chronic idiopathic constipation [53, 54]. Given the benefits of other 5-HT_4 agonists for the treatment of CIC and IBS-C, naronapride has the potential to improve symptoms in FGID patients.

Brain-Gut Axis and the Gut Microbiome

As mentioned earlier, a key component of the brain-gut axis is the lumen of the GI tract and its contents. The contents include the gut microbiome, the incredibly rich, complicated, and delicately balanced ecosystem now recognized to play an intimate role in the brain-gut axis. For example, experimental alterations in the gut flora of germ-free mice can inhibit an exaggerated release of corticosterone and ACTH in response to stress [55]. As well, the combination of 2 different probiotics (*Lactobacillus helveticus* R0052 and *Bifidobacterium longum* R0157) reduces anxiety in rats [56]. Conversely, the brain can influence the microbiome. Adult rats separated early at birth from their mother had a change in the fecal microbiome (using 16S rRNA analysis) compared to those rats not subjected to maternal separation [57]. Although beyond the scope of this chapter, it is easy to imagine how prebiotics, probiotics, antibiotics, prokinetics, and diet could all contribute to changes in the gut microbiome, and thus influence CNS function via the brain-gut axis.

Conclusion

FGIDs are highly prevalent heterogeneous group of disorders characterized by recurrent GI symptoms in the absence of endoscopic, radiographic, or biochemical abnormality. Despite their high prevalence, treatment options have been sparse, and efficacy has been limited. This is in part due to the inherent limitations of medications that only target the wall and lumen of the GI tract. The brain-gut axis is dynamic and is composed of the CNS, ENS, hypothalamus-pituitary-adrenal axis, and the gut microbiota, in addition to the wall and lumen of the GI tract. Recognizing the complex relationship between coexisting psychosocial conditions such as anxiety, depression, and somatization in many patients with FGIDs, the brain-gut axis represents a perfect target for medical and psychological therapies. This broad approach, targeting the brain-gut axis and its complex interplay of different systems, may eventually prove most fruitful in the treatment of FGIDs.

References

1 Locke GR, Talley NJ, Fett SL, et al: Prevalence and clinical spectrum of gastroesophageal reflux: a population-based study in Olmsted County, Minnesota. Gastroenterology 1997;112:1448–1456.
2 Drossman DA, Li Z, Andruzzi E, Temple RD, et al: U.S. householder survey of functional gastrointestinal disorders. Prevalence, sociodemography, and health impact. Dig Dis Sci 1993;38:1569–1580.
3 Webster R, Norman P, Goodacre S, et al: The prevalence and correlates of psychological outcomes in patients with acute non-cardiac chest pain: a systematic review. Emerg Med J 2012;29:267–273.
4 Richter JE, Bradley LA, Castell DO: Esophageal chest pain: current controversies in pathogenesis, diagnosis, and therapy. Ann Intern Med 1989;110: 66–78.
5 Hershcovici T, Achem SR, Jha LK, et al: Systematic review: the treatment of noncardiac chest pain. Aliment Pharmacol Ther 2012;35:5–14.
6 Holzer P: Acid-sensitive ion channels in gastrointestinal function. Curr Opin Pharmacol 2003;3:618–625.
7 Krarup AL, Ny L, Gunnarsson J, et al: Randomized clinical trial: inhibition of the TRPV1 system in patients with nonerosive gastroesophageal reflux disease and a partial response to PPI treatment is not associated with analgesia to esophageal experimental pain. Scand J Gastroenterol 2013;48:274–284.
8 Sarkar S, Hobson AR, Hughes A, et al: The prostaglandin E2 receptor-1 (EP-1) mediates acid-induced visceral pain hypersensitivity in humans. Gastroenterology 2003;124:18–25.
9 Kondo T, Oshima T, Tomita T, et al: Prostaglandin E2 mediates acid-induced heartburn in healthy volunteers. Am J Physiol Gastrointest Liver Physiol 2013;304:G568–G573.
10 Hornby PJ, Prouty SM: Involvement of cannabinoid receptors in gut motility and visceral perception. Br J Pharmacol 2004;141:1335–1345.
11 Jones H, Cooper P, Miller V, et al: Treatment of noncardiac chest pain: a controlled trial of hypnotherapy. Gut 2006;55:1403–1408.
12 Vakil N, van Zanten SV, Kahrilas P, et al: The Montreal definition and classification of gastroesophageal reflux disease: a global evidence-based consensus. Am J Gastroenterol 2006;101:1900–1920.
13 Dent J, El-Serag HB, Wallander MA, et al: Epidemiology of gastro-oesophageal reflux disease: a systematic review. Gut 2005;54:710–717.
14 Camilleri M, Dubois D, Coulie B, et al: Prevalence and socioeconomic impact of upper gastrointestinal disorders in the United States: results of the US Upper Gastrointestinal Study. Clin Gastroenterol Hepatol 2005;3:543–552.
15 Eslick GD, Talley NJ: Gastroesophageal reflux disease (GERD): risk factors, and impact on quality of life – a population-based study. J Clin Gastroenterol 2009;43:111–117.
16 Becher A, El-Serag H: Systematic review: the association between symptomatic response to proton pump inhibitors and health-related quality of life in patients with gastro-oesophageal reflux disease. Aliment Pharmacol Ther 2011;34:618–627.

17 Vakil NB, Huff FJ, Bian A, et al: Arbaclofen placarbil in GERD: a randomized, double-blind, placebo-controlled study. Am J Gastroenterol 2011;106:1427–1438.
18 Zerbib F, Bruley des Varannes S, Roman S, et al: Randomised clinical trial: effects of monotherapy with ADX10059, a mGluR5 inhibitor, on symptoms and reflux events in patients with gastro-oesophageal reflux disease. Aliment Pharmacol Ther 2011;33:911–921.
19 Lidums I, Lehmann A, Checklin H, et al: Control of transient lower esophageal sphincter relaxations and reflux by the GABA(B) agonist baclofen in normal subjects. Gastroenterology 2000;118:7–13.
20 Kahrilas PJ, Quigley EM, Castell DO, et al: The effects of tegaserod (HTF 919) on oesophageal acid exposure in gastro-oesophageal reflux disease. Aliment Pharmacol Ther 2000;14:1503–1509.
21 Altan E, Masaoka T, Farré R, et al: Acotiamide, a novel gastroprokinetic for the treatment of patients with functional dyspepsia: postprandial distress syndrome. Expert Rev Gastroenterol Hepatol 2012;6:533–534.
22 Kusunoki H, Haruma K, Manabe N, et al: Therapeutic efficacy of acotiamide in patients with functional dyspepsia based on enhanced postprandial gastric accommodation and emptying: randomized controlled study evaluation by real-time ultrasonography. Neurogastroenterol Motil 2012;24:540–545.
23 Matsueda K, Hongo M, Tack J, et al: A placebo-controlled trial of acotiamide for meal-related symptoms of functional dyspepsia. Gut 2012;61:821–828.
24 Johnston JM, Shiff SJ, Quigley EM: A review of the clinical efficacy of linaclotide in irritable bowel syndrome with constipation. Curr Med Res Opin 2013;29:149–160.
25 Eutamene H, Bradesi S, Larauche M, et al: Guanylate cyclase C-mediated antinociceptive effects of linaclotide in rodent models of visceral pain. Neurogastroenterol Motil 2010;22:312-e84.
26 Fukuda H, Mizuta Y, Isomoto H, et al: Ghrelin enhances gastric motility through direct stimulation of intrinsic neural pathways and capsaicin-sensitive afferent neurons in rats. Scand J Gastroenterol 2004;39:1209–1214.
27 Murray CD, Martin NM, Patterson M, et al: Ghrelin enhances gastric emptying in diabetic gastroparesis: a double-blind, placebo-controlled, crossover study. Gut 2005;54:1693–1698.
28 Tack J, Depoortere I, Bisschops R, et al: Influence of ghrelin on gastric emptying and meal-related symptoms in idiopathic gastroparesis. Aliment Pharmacol Ther 2005;22:847–853.
29 Ejskjaer N, Wo JM, Esfandyari T, et al: A phase 2a, randomized, double-blind 28-day study of TZP-102 a ghrelin receptor agonist for diabetic gastroparesis. Neurogastroenterol Motil 2013;25:e140–e150.
30 Trudel L, Tomasetto C, Rio MC, et al: Ghrelin/motilin-related peptide is a potent prokinetic to reverse gastric postoperative ileus in rat. Am J Physiol Gastrointest Liver Physiol 2002;282:G948–G952.
31 Jackson JL, O'Malley PG, Tomkins G, et al: Treatment of functional gastrointestinal disorders with antidepressant medications: a meta-analysis. Am J Med 2002;108:65–72.
32 Lesbros-Pantoflickova D, Michetti P, Fried M, et al: Meta-analysis: the treatment of irritable bowel syndrome. Aliment Pharmacol Ther 2004;20:1253–1269.
33 Drossman DA, Toner BB, Whitehead WE, et al: Cognitive-behavioral therapy versus education and desipramine versus placebo for moderate to severe functional bowel disorders. Gastroenterology 2003;125:19–31.
34 Tabas G, Beaves M, Wang J, et al: Paroxetine to treat irritable bowel syndrome not responding to high-fiber diet. Am J Gastroenterol 2004;99:914–920.
35 Masand PS, Gupta S, Schwartz TL, et al: Paroxetine in patients with irritable bowel syndrome; a pilot open-label study. Prim Care Companion J Clin Psychiatry 2002;4:12–16.
36 Vahedi H, Merat S, Rashidioon A, et al: The effect of fluoxetine on patients with pain and constipation predominant irritable bowel syndrome; a double-blind, randomized-controlled study. Aliment Pharmacol Ther 2005;22:381–385.
37 Kuiken SD, Tytgat GN, Boeckxstaens GE: The selective serotonin reuptake inhibitor fluoxetine does not change rectal sensitivity and symptoms in patients with irritable bowel syndrome; a double-blind, randomized, placebo-controlled study. Clin Gastroenterol Hepatol 2003;3:219–228.
38 Tack J, Broekaert D, Fischler B, et al: A controlled crossover study of the selective serotonin reuptake inhibitor citalopram in irritable bowel syndrome. Gut 2006;55:1095–1103.
39 Talley NJ, Kellow JE, Boyce P, et al: Antidepressant therapy (imipramine and citalopram) for irritable bowel syndrome: a double blind, randomized, placebo-controlled trial. Dig Dis Sci 2008;53:108–115.
40 Ford AC, Talley NJ, Schoenfeld PS, et al: Efficacy of antidepressants and psychological therapies in irritable bowel syndrome: systematic review and meta-analysis. Gut DOI:10.1136/gut.2008.163162.
41 Clouse RE: Antidepressants for irritable bowel syndrome. Gut 2003;52:598–599.
42 Brennan BP, Fogarty KV, Roberts JL, et al: Duloxetine in the treatment of irritable bowel syndrome: an open-label pilot study. Hum Psychopharmacol 2009;24:423–428.
43 Gale JD, Houghton LA: Alpha 2 delta (α2δ) ligands, gabapentin and pregabalin: what is the evidence for potential use of these ligands in irritable bowel syndrome. Front Pharmacol 2011;2:1–9.

44 Lee KJ, Kim JH, Cho SW: Gabepentin reduces rectal mechanosensitivity and increases rectal compliance in patients with diarrhea-predominant irritable bowel syndrome. Aliment Pharmacol Ther 2005;22: 981–988.
45 Houghton LA, Fell C, Whorwell P, et al: Effect of a second generation α2δ ligand (pregabalin) on visceral sensation in hypersensitive patients with irritable bowel syndrome. Gut 2007;56:1218–1225.
46 Leventer SM, Raudibaugh K, Frissora CL, Kassem N, Keogh JC, Phillips J, et al: Clinical trial: dextofisopam in the treatment of patients with diarrhoea-predominant or alternating irritable bowel syndrome. Aliment Pharmacol Ther 2008;27:197–206.
47 Delvaux M, Beck A, Jacob J, Bouzamondo H, Weber FT, Frexinos J: Effect of asimadoline, a kappa opioid agonist, on pain induced by colonic distention in patients with irritable bowel syndrome. Aliment Pharmacol Ther 2004;20:237–246.
48 Mangel AW, Bornstein JD, Hamm LR, et al: Clinical trial: asimadoline in the treatment of patients with irritable bowel syndrome. Aliment Pharmacol Ther 2008;28:239–249.
49 Gershon MD, Tack J: The serotonin signaling system: from basic understanding to drug development for functional GI disorders. Gastroenterology 2007; 132:397–414.
50 Zambrowicz B, Brown PM, Drossman DA, et al: 5-HT biomarker levels correlate with clinical response in phase 2 trial of LX1031, a novel 5-HT synthesis inhibitor for non-constipating IBS. Gastroenterology 2009;136(suppl 1):S168.
51 Tillisch K, Labus J, Nam B, et al: Neurokinin-1-receptor antagonism decreases anxiety and emotional arousal circuit response to noxious visceral distention in women with irritable bowel syndrome: a pilot study. Aliment Pharmacol Ther 2012;35:360–367.
52 Bowersox SS, Lightning LK, Rao S, et al: Metabolism and pharmacokinetics of naronapride (ATI-7505), a serotonin 5-HT4 receptor agonist for gastrointestinal motility disorders. Drug Metabol Disposition 2011;39:1170–1180.
53 Camilleri M, Vazquez-Roque MI, Burton D, et al: Pharmacodynamic effects of a novel prokinetic 5-HT4 receptor agonist, ATI-7505, in humans. Neurogastroenterol Motil 2007;19:30–38.
54 Palme M, Milner P, Randman O, et al: A novel gastrointestinal prokinetic ATI-7505 increased spontaneous bowel movements in a phase II randomized, placebo-controlled study of patients with chronic idiopathic constipation. Gastroenterology 2010; 138(suppl 1):S128–S129.
55 Sudo N, Chia Y, Aiba Y, et al: Postnatal microbial colonization programs the hypothalamic-pituitary-adrenal system for stress response in mice. J Physiol (London) 2004;558:263–275.
56 Messaoudi M, Lalonde R, Violle N, et al: Assessment of psychotropic-like properties of a probiotic formulation (*Lactobacillus helveticus* R0052 and *Bifidobacterium longum* R0175) in rats and human subjects. Br J Nutr 2011;105:755–764.
57 O'Mahony SM, Marchesi JR, Scully P, et al: Early life stress alters behavior, immunity, and microbiota in rats: implications for irritable bowel syndrome and psychiatric illnesses. Biol Psychiatry 2009;65:263–267.
58 Mayer EA, Tillisch K: The brain-gut axis in abdominal pain syndromes. Annu Rev Med 2011;62:381–396.

Scott Gabbard, MD
Division of Gastroenterology and Hepatology, Dartmouth-Hitchcock Medical Center
1 Medical Center Drive
Lebanon, NH 03756 (USA)
E-Mail gabbars@ccf.org

Quigley EMM, Hongo M, Fukudo S (eds): Functional and GI Motility Disorders.
Front Gastrointest Res. Basel, Karger, 2014, vol 33, pp 130–140 (DOI: 10.1159/000356985)

Specific Clinical Contexts – Part 1: The Intensive Care Unit

Eamonn M.M. Quigley
Division of Gastroenterology, The Methodist Hospital, Houston, Tex., USA

Abstract
The acutely ill patient who requires admission to the intensive care unit is at risk for a number of potentially life-threatening disorders of gut motility. Predisposing and/or precipitating factors may include the underlying illness itself, recent surgery, sepsis and a variety of medications. As these patients are often heavily sedated or unconscious, the development of these motility problems may be silent and not become clinically obvious until complications have developed, necessitating that the clinician be ever alert for their presence. Among the various motility syndromes that have been described in this context, megacolon is, perhaps, the most common. When detected, a number of therapeutic options are available for the management of megacolon, depending on its severity and rate of development. While aspiration and feeding difficulties are well-known challenges in the intensive care unit, their pathophysiology has been poorly understood. Studies of upper gastrointestinal motor function have demonstrated that the critically ill are subject to profound alterations in motor and sensory function of the esophagus, lower esophageal sphincter, stomach and duodenum which go some way towards explaining their propensity to reflux and gastroparesis, with their attendant risks. New data on the pathogenesis of postoperative ileus may throw light on ICU-related dysmotility, in general, and open some new therapeutic avenues. Indeed, recent studies have identified a number of strategies and new pharmacological approaches to the management of postoperative ileus which have the potential to be used in the nonsurgical ICU patient.

As more and more patients are subjected to surgical procedures of increasing complexity and risk and as survival rates from catastrophic illnesses rise, due to advances in surgery, anesthesia and intensive care, one would expect an associated growth in awareness of, and research into, the effects of critical illness on gut motor function. While a considerable literature exists on the pathophysiology and management of postoperative ileus, motor function and dysfunction in the nonsurgical ICU patient have received relatively attention, and our understanding of the factors which contribute to dysmotility in this patient population and of strategies to alleviate it are far less well developed. While a high prevalence, in the critically ill patient, of such phenomena as gastroesophageal reflux and gastroparesis are assumed, their true rates of occurrence have been scarcely documented. Similarly, while potential consequences of these entities, such as aspiration, esophagitis, nosocomial pneumonia, feeding difficulties and even gastric perforation are well known and, justifiably, feared, the effects of critical illness on esophageal and gastric motor function have been little investigated.

There are, it must be conceded, many reasons for this. Several factors, intrinsic to any intensive care (or therapy) unit patient population, deter the clinician-scientist from embarking on the investigation of these subjects and confound the interpretation of any studies completed. First and foremost, this is, by definition, a heterogeneous population. Depending on the nature of a particular unit, it may include, among its patients, a wide range of ages, as well as a diverse catalog of precipitating illnesses and events. Among the latter, prior surgery, raised intracranial pressure, intraabdominal or systemic sepsis, cranial, abdominal or spinal trauma and such conditions as acute pancreatitis and intestinal ischemia will directly influence gut motor function. Within each of these categories, further heterogeneity prevails; ileus following surgery being especially prevalent in relation, not only to extensive abdominal procedures, but also to abdominal aortic, cardiac and spinal surgery [1]. Preexisting illnesses, such as diabetes, cardiac failure or renal insufficiency (ever more present in the modern ICU population) will also influence the response to acute stress and the likelihood of motor dysfunction. Electrolyte abnormalities are common in the critically ill and can influence the function of excitable tissues, including intestinal nerve and muscle.

Secondly, these patients are prey to a host of iatrogenic influences on gut motor function. The typical ICU patient receives significant sedation and analgesia, often requires mechanical ventilation, commonly receives adrenergic agents for circulatory support and relies on either total parenteral (TPN) or enteral nutritional support: all can influence gut motor function. The administration of TPN, together with the metabolic effects of acute stress, may result in significant fluctuations in blood sugar levels with their attendant effects on gut, and especially gastric motility. Hyperglycemia, for example, can profoundly suppress gastric motility and delay gastric emptying rate. Enhanced glucose absorption and hyperglycemia have been well documented among the critically ill, and while hyperglycemia has been identified as a significant predictor of adverse outcomes, it must be noted that these patients are also prone to develop hypoglycemia with intensive insulin therapy [2].

Finally, these patients are critically ill and rarely fully conscious. Symptoms cannot be expressed, thereby, ensuring that the consequences of motor dysfunction will be,

Table 1. Factors contributing to gut motor dysfunction in the ICU patient

Premorbid conditions (e.g. diabetes, renal insufficiency, hypothyroidism, cardiac failure)
Recent surgery
Head injury
Raised intracranial pressure
Fluid overload
Electrolyte imbalance
Hyperglycemia
Fasting
Medications
Opiates
Vasopressors
Sepsis
Peritonitis
Intraabdominal hemorrhage
Pancreatitis

for the most part, silent. These same factors may give rise to difficulties in relation to consent and ability to cooperate with research protocols.

Some insight into the prevalence of gastrointestinal problems in the ICU patient was provided by Reintam et al. [3] who retrospectively reviewed the incidence of what they termed 'gastrointestinal failure' among over 2,500 patients in three ICUs in Germany and Estonia. 'Gastrointestinal failure', a catch-all term that included clinically overt gastrointestinal hemorrhage, ileus and food intolerance, occurred in almost 10% of all patients and was associated with increased mortality, longer stays in the ICU and more prolonged periods of mechanical ventilation. Disease severity, presence of multiorgan failure and the use of vasopressors were predictors of the development of 'gastrointestinal failure'. However, studies which more directly assessed motor function have suggested a much higher prevalence of dysmotility with, for example, impaired gastric emptying being described in 50–80% [2, 4, 5]. Constipation was reported, in one study, in 70% of 106 nonsurgical ICU patients [6]. While none of the usual factors were predictive of constipation, early enteral feeding was protective against its development.

Pathogenesis of Gut Motor Dysfunction in the ICU Patient

Several patient and clinical factors are known to contribute to the pathogenesis of gut motor dysfunction in the ICU patient and are listed in table 1 [2, 4, 5]. Among surgical procedures, certain operations are known to confer particular risk, such as major open abdominal procedures, as well as cardiac, spinal and aortic surgery. It is now abundantly evident that laparoscopic procedures are associated with a more rapid return of gut motor function than their open equivalents, with motility returning a day earlier, on average. Recent research has emphasized the importance of the inflammatory response in the pathogenesis of postoperative ileus and, indeed, of gut motor dysfunction, in general, in the postoperative patient [7–11]. According to this hypothesis, inflammation of the muscle layers of the gut is the basic mechanism of postoperative ileus. This inflammatory response is initiated by handling and other traumas to the intestine that trigger the release of inflammatory cytokines and the expression of adhesion molecules on endothelial cells [11]. This, in turn, promotes the migration of monocytes into the muscularis [7] and they, together with resident macrophages, produce nitric oxide [8] and prostaglandins; both are inhibitory to gut motility. These immunological responses can result in ileus throughout the gastrointestinal tract [10]. That these mechanisms might also apply to the nonsurgical ICU patient seems plausible as other factors (sepsis and pancreatitis, for example) in such individuals, could generate similar inflammatory responses. Needless to say, this concept opens the way to new therapeutic strategies such as the use of cyclooxygenase 2 (COX-2) inhibitors, monoclonal antibodies against adhesion molecules, glycine (for its immunomodulatory effects), mast cell stabilizers and matrix metalloproteinase inhibitors [11].

Prevention

In comprehensive reviews of the modern approach to postoperative ileus, van Bree et al. [11] and Johnson and Walsh [12] listed several clinical factors which can reduce the risk of ileus in the postoperative patient:

1 Perioperative factors
  a Fluid and electrolyte management (avoiding fluid overload and electrolyte abnormalities)
  b Early ambulation
  c Optimal analgesia
2 Use of laparoscopic rather than open approaches to abdominal surgery
3 Epidural local anesthetics
4 Laxatives
5 Positioning and movement of the patient in the bed to promote colonic gas expulsion

Several pharmacological approaches have been taken to the prevention of postoperative ileus. The peripheral μ-opioid receptor antagonist alvimopan was shown to be effective but was associated with an increased rate of myocardial infarction [13]. Traditional prokinetics, though potentially useful in therapy, were not effective in preventing ileus when evaluated in a Cochrane systematic review [14]. However, newer, more specific 5-HT_4 agonists, such as prucalopride and mosapride, may, however, be effective [15]. Clinical studies have also shown promise for parenteral lidocaine [16], epidural neostigmine [17], subcutaneous methylnaltrexone [18], ghrelin agonists and

COX-2 inhibitors [11]. Again, it must be stressed that these studies were confined to postoperative ileus; the extent to which their findings can be extrapolated to ileus, in general, is not known.

Esophageal Dysfunction and Gastroparesis

Prevalence

While acute gastroparesis is a well-known, potentially disastrous, but relatively rare complication of acute illness, the gastroenterologist is more likely to be consulted regarding the potential contributions of dysmotility to more common but, perhaps, less obvious manifestations of gastroparesis: feeding problems, increased gastric residues, reflux and aspiration. Increased gastric residual volumes (variably defined as >150 ml) have been directly correlated with delayed gastric emptying [19]; this is, perhaps, the most commonly detected manifestation of intolerance to enteral feeding, a complication that has been reported in up to 50% of ICU patients [2]. Furthermore, Nind et al. [20] described the presence of gastroesophageal reflux in 60% of ICU patients.

Pathophysiology

Recent investigations have provided some important insights into gastric and esophageal function in the critically ill. Taken together, these studies provide some striking and clinically important observations on foregut motility in the critically ill; when combined, they provide a frightening scenario which goes some way to explaining the prevalence of feeding intolerance and aspiration in this patient population.

Turning, firstly, to their studies of esophageal motor function [20]. Among fifteen mechanically ventilated patients, using simultaneous measurements of esophageal motility, impedance and intraluminal pH, they documented some striking abnormalities. Lower esophageal sphincter (LES) pressure was virtually nonexistent (averaging just 2.2 mm Hg!) and the motor response to reflux (secondary peristalsis) was strikingly impaired. Not surprisingly, reflux was frequent and often prolonged; in some patients, pH was below 4 for the entire 6-hour study period. The median percentage of time that pH was below 4 was 39% during fasting and 32% following nutrient administration. Reflux events were related to either absent LES pressure or the occurrence of straining, on a background of marked LES hypotension. Most episodes of straining were precipitated by coughing; in turn, usually provoked by endotracheal tube suction, a familiar scenario in any ICU. The ICU patient is clearly at extreme risk for acid reflux, whose prevalence must have been greatly underestimated in the past if these data are in any way representative of the general ICU population. Acid may not be the only risk factor. In the ICU, parenteral acid suppression has become the norm; in this hypo- or achlorhydric environment bacterial overgrowth may occur in the stomach [21] and could, through nonacid reflux events, lead to the development of aspiration pneumonia. Furthermore, one could speculate that therapy directed at the LES or esophageal body function, may, ultimately, prove to be more appropriate than acid suppression in the ICU.

In their other studies, involving the stomach and duodenum, the findings were equally alarming [22–24]. Fifteen mechanically ventilated ICU patients were subjected to antro-pyloro-duodenal manometry and gastric emptying in the fasted state and following intragastric and intraduodenal nutrient infusion at the very modest rate of 1 kcal/min [22]. The most striking finding was the profound inhibition of antral motility that resulted from either intragastric or intraduodenal nutrient installation; a similar rate of nutrient infusion to healthy volunteers had no effect on this parameter of gastric motor function. Intraduodenal nutrient also provoked isolated pyloric pressure waves and augmented pyloric tone, phenomena which would serve to further impair gastric emptying. Gastric emptying, was, not surprisingly, delayed. Taken together, these findings indicate a profound 'upregulation' of the feedback loop which normally regulates the gastric emptying of nutrients and guarantees the steady delivery of 2–3 kcal/min to the small intestine, thus ensuring optimal digestive function. In the ICU patient, this very same mechanism appears to be preventing the egress of gastric contents in response to a duodenal nutrient delivery rate of just 1 kcal/min, an observation that may go some way towards explaining the frequency of intolerance to enteral nutrition in this population. In a more detailed examination of antroduodenal motility, they subsequently described how coordination between antral and duodenal motor events, so critical to efficient gastric delivery of nutrients in health, was severely disrupted in the critically ill patient [23]. Furthermore, nutrient-induced gastric relaxation is impaired in the proximal stomach, and coordination between the proximal and distal stomach is lost [24], resulting in abnormal distribution of the meal within the stomach.

Though these studies carefully controlled for some of the factors that have bedeviled prior investigations, the pathophysiology of these esophageal and gastric motor changes remain unclear and the relative contributions of such factors as underlying illness, mechanical ventilation or hypotension remain unresolved. By invoking an abnormality in the intestinal sensing of nutrient, one of these studies does indicate that, in terms of gastric function, the primary abnormality may not be simple 'pump' failure, as has been described by others in the critically ill [25–27], but rather a hypersensitive intestine-gastric feedback loop.

Regardless of the pathogenesis of these findings, everyone who cares for these patients must be aware of the triple jeopardy to which these patients are prone: LES hypotension, esophageal body dysmotility and gastroparesis. When combined, these factors expose the ICU patient to an extreme risk of aspiration of acid or, alternately, pathogen-enriched, acid-depleted gastric juice. These findings demand that we pay much more care and attention to motor dysfunction and the delivery of enteral nutrition to a highly vulnerable patient population.

Management

Apart from the general measures described above, some specific approaches may be indicated in the ICU patient with upper GI dysmotility. If feeding intolerance is the main manifestation, alternative feeding routes may be instituted. A recent meta-analysis reviewed the impact on the positioning of an enteral feeding tube on various outcomes. In comparison to intragastric feeding, small bowel feeding was associated with improved nutrient intake and a reduced risk of pneumonia, but duration of ventilation, length of ICU stay and mortality were unaffected by the route of feeding [28]. In contrast, in a multicenter study from Australia and New Zealand, nasojejunal feeding did not confer any clinical advantage over nasogastric feeding among patients with mildly increased gastric residuals [29]. Despite their poor results in prevention, metoclopramide and erythromycin have been shown in some, but not all, studies to improve clinically relevant parameters of gastric function in this population [4]. Tolerance is a real problem with erythromycin, and concerns have also been raised about its potential to promote antibiotic resistance in a population at high risk of sepsis [30].

Ileus and Small Intestinal Motility

For obvious reasons, small intestinal motility has been rarely studied in this population. In recordings from the proximal small intestine, among critically ill patients, duodenal motility was disrupted with a failure to convert to a fed pattern and a persistence of burst activity, hardly the ideal accompaniment for the digestive process [22]. These observations also illustrate how small intestinal dysmotility can contribute to feeding intolerance. Stasis in the small intestine coupled with impaired intestinal barrier function and immunosuppression (all known accompaniments of critical illness) are thought to conspire in leading to small intestinal bacterial overgrowth, bacterial translocation and systemic sepsis and even multiorgan failure syndrome [31]. However, the impact of strategies to promote intestinal transit, modulate the microbiota (by intestinal decontamination, antibiotics, prebiotics, or probiotics) or improve barrier function, while promising in experimental studies have not been consistently successful in the clinical context, and a detailed discussion of their role is beyond the scope of this review [32]. One intervention does appear to promote epithelial integrity and immune function: enteral nutrition [32].

Megacolon, Ogilvie's Syndrome

Definition and Etiology

Acute colonic pseudo-obstruction, or Ogilvie's syndrome, is defined as an acute dilatation of the colon without evidence of mechanical obstruction distal to the dilated segment [33]. Ogilvie's syndrome is associated with an underlying medical condition or the postoperative state in over 90% of cases. Risk factors for the development of Ogilvie's syndrome in individual patients following surgery include: advanced age, obesity, immobility, and use of patient-controlled analgesia.

Clinical Presentation

Progressive abdominal distention is the clinical hallmark of this condition; in the postoperative state, distention is, typically, evident by the 4th postoperative day. Lower abdominal pain and nausea and vomiting are present in 60–80 and 50%, respectively. It is important to realize that, while the vast majority of patients with Ogilvie's syndrome are completely constipated, megacolon can develop in individuals who continue to pass both stool and flatus. Only 40% of patients will have hypoactive or absent bowel sounds. The overall risk of perforation in Ogilvie's syndrome is low, in the region of 3%, but mortality following perforation, in this context, may be as high as 50%. Cecal diameter is valuable in predicting risk of perforation; a diameter in excess of 9 cm is abnormal, and when greater than 12 cm, indicates a significant risk of perforation.

Differential Diagnosis

In the patient with acute megacolon, the main differential diagnoses to be considered are, firstly, toxic megacolon and, secondly, acute colonic obstruction due to carcinoma, benign (e.g. diverticular) stricture, volvulus or intussusception.

Toxic megacolon should be obvious from the patient's history and clinical presentation, and obstruction may be suspected by the prominence of pain in the symptomatology, as well as by clinical and radiographic findings. It is important to note that, on X-ray, haustral markings are preserved in Ogilvie's syndrome, in contrast to both toxic megacolon and obstruction.

Diagnostic Methods

Plain abdominal X-ray may be the only essential investigation. Typically, there is dilatation of the cecum and ascending and transverse colon with less gaseous distention in the left colon. If obstruction needs to be ruled out, computerized abdominal tomography may, nowadays, be the best option with barium enema and colonoscopy as alternatives. If colonoscopy is contemplated, the endoscopist needs to be mindful of the risk of a cecal perforation due to the closed loop phenomenon, if obstruction is complete.

Management

The first step in the management of acute megacolon is to search for and, where possible, treat any underlying disorder. Many cases will resolve spontaneously as the associated primary disorder improves; frequent changes in patient position may also promote resolution. In resistant cases, therapy should begin with a pharmacological approach.

Cholinergic agonists are effective. Ponec et al. [33] administered neostigmine in a dose of 2 mg intravenously to 11 patients with acute colonic pseudo-obstruction and compared their outcome with that of 10 who received intravenous saline. Ten of the 11 patients who received neostigmine had prompt colonic decompression compared with none of the 10 patients who received placebo. The median time for response was 4 min. Two patients who had an initial response to neostigmine required colonoscopic decompression for recurrence of colonic distention; one eventually underwent subtotal colectomy. In contrast, 7 patients in the placebo group and one patient in the neostigmine group without an initial response received open-label neostigmine; all achieved colonic decompression. Subsequent, uncontrolled and retrospective studies, which involved the administration of neostigmine by either intravenous infusion or an intravenous bolus, have confirmed the efficacy of neostigmine with response rates ranging from 61 to 100% [34, 35]. Bradycardia was the most significant side effect of neostigmine, occurring in 7.2% overall and appeared to be more common when administered by bolus injection; for this reason, cardiac monitoring is recommended, especially in high-risk individuals. It is important to emphasize that only one of these studies [36] was a prospective, randomized, placebo-controlled trial [34, 35].

Given the risk of spontaneous perforation with its associated high mortality, colonoscopy has played an important role in the management of patients with megacolon and significant cecal distention [35, 37]. By definition, the colon will not be prepared in these patients, and the procedure may, therefore, be technically difficult. Colonoscopy should be reserved for those who fail conservative therapy, including neostigmine, in view of its risks in Ogilvie's syndrome. An overall success rate, in achieving a reduction in cecal diameter, of 61–70% has been reported with a first colonoscopy; this success rate rises to 73–88% after one or more procedures. However, the recurrence rate has been approximately 40% [38]. Uncontrolled data suggest that this may be decreased with the placement of a decompression tube at the time of colonoscopy. This involves the placement of a guide-wire through the biopsy channel of the colonoscope with the subsequent insertion of the decompression tube over the guide-wire, under fluoroscopic control, following withdrawal of the colonoscope [39].

Surgical intervention and the placement of a tube cecostomy, in particular, may become necessary in the patient with megacolon who appears at high risk of perforation and has failed pharmacological and colonoscopic attempts at decompression. Clearly, surgery will also be necessary in those who unfortunately progress to ischemia or perforation. In all of these situations, surgery has been associated with high morbidity and mortality rates, in the region of 30 and 6%, respectively [38].

References

1 Quigley EMM: Acute intestinal pseudo-obstruction. Curr Treat Options Gastroenterol 2000;3:273–285.
2 Deane A, Chapman MJ, Fraser RJL, Horowitz M: Bench-to-bedside review: the gut as an endocrine organ in the critically ill. Crit Care 2010;14:228.
3 Reintam A, Parm P, Redlich U, Tooding LM, Starkopf J, Köhler F, Spies C, Kern H: Gastrointestinal failure in intensive care: a retrospective clinical study in three different intensive care units in Germany and Estonia. BMC Gastroenterol 2006;6:19.
4 Stupak DP, Abdelsayed GG, Soloway GN: Motility disorders of the upper gastrointestinal tract in the intensive care unit. Pathophysiology and contemporary management. J Clin Gastroenterol 2012;46:449–456.
5 Fruhwald S, Holzer P, Metzler H: Intestinal motility disturbances in intensive care patients pathogenesis and clinical impact. Intensive Care Med 2007;33:36–44.
6 Nassar AP Jr, Queiroz de Silva FM, de Cleva R: Constipation in intensive care unit: incidence and risk factors. J Crit Care 2009;24:630e9–630e12.
7 Kalff JC, Carlos TM, Schraut WH, Billiar TR, Simmons RL, Bauer AJ: Surgically induced leukocytic infiltrates within the rat intestinal muscularis mediate postoperative ileus. Gastroenterology 1999;117:378–387.
8 Kalff JC, Schraut WH, Billiar TR, Simmons RL, Bauer AJ: Role of inducible nitric oxide synthase in postoperative intestinal smooth muscle dysfunction in rodents. Gastroenterology 2000;118:316–327.
9 Luckey A, Livingston E, Taché Y: Mechanisms and treatment of postoperative ileus. Arch Surg 2003; 138:206–214.
10 Engel DR, Koscielny A, Wehner S, Maurer J, Schiwon M, Franken L, Schumak B, Limmer A, Sparwasser T, Hirner A, Knolle PA, Kalff JC, Kurts C: T helper type 1 memory cells disseminate postoperative ileus over the entire intestinal tract. Nat Med 2010;16:1407–1413.
11 Van Bree SHW, Nemethova A, Cailotto C, Gomez-Pinilla PJ, Matteoli G, Boeckxstaens GE: New therapeutic strategies for postoperative ileus. Nat Rev Gastroenterol Hepatol 2012;9:675–683.
12 Johnson MD, Walsh RM: Current therapies to shorten postoperative ileus. Cleveland Clin J Med 2009; 76:641–648.
13 Ludwig K, Viscusi ER, Wolff BG, Delaney CP, Senagore A, Techner L: Alvimopan for the management of postoperative ileus after bowel resection: characterization of clinical benefit by pooled responder analysis. World J Surg 2010;34:2185–2190.
14 Traut U, Brügger L, Kunz R, Pauli-Magnus C, Haug K, Bucher HC, Koller MT: Systemic prokinetic pharmacologic treatment for postoperative adynamic ileus following abdominal surgery in adults. Cochrane Database Syst Rev 2008;(1):CD004930.
15 Quigley EM: Prucalopride: safety, efficacy and potential applications. Therap Adv Gastroenterol 2012; 5:23–30.
16 Herroeder S, Pecher S, Schönherr ME, Kaulitz G, Hahnenkamp K, Friess H, Böttiger BW, Bauer H, Dijkgraaf MG, Durieux ME, Hollmann MW: Systemic lidocaine shortens length of hospital stay after colorectal surgery: a double-blinded, randomized, placebo-controlled trial. Ann Surg 2007;246:192–200.
17 Caliskan E, Turkoz A, Sener M, Bozdogan N, Gulcan O, Turkoz R: A prospective randomized double-blind study to determine the effect of thoracic epidural neostigmine on postoperative ileus after abdominal aortic surgery. Anesth Analg 2008;106: 959–964.
18 Sawh SB, Selvaraj IP, Danga A, Cotton AL, Moss J, Patel PB: Use of methylnaltrexone for the treatment of opioid-induced constipation in critical care patients. Mayo Clin Proc 2012;87:255–259.
19 Landzinski J, Kiser TH, Fish DN, Wischmeyer PE, MacLaren R: Gastric motility function in critically ill patients tolerant vs intolerant to gastric nutrition. JPEN 2008;32:45–50.
20 Nind G, Chen WH, Protheroe R, Iwakiri K, Fraser R, Young R, Chapman M, Nguyen N, Sifrim D, Rigda R, Holloway RH: Mechanisms of gastroesophageal reflux in critically ill mechanically ventilated patients. Gastroenterology 2005;128:600–606.
21 Williams C: Occurrence and significance of gastric colonization during acid-inhibitory therapy. Best Pract Res Clin Gastroenterol 2001;15:511–521.
22 Chapman M, Fraser R, Vozzo R, Bryant L, Tam W, Nguyen N, Zacharakis B, Butler R, Davidson G, Horowitz M: Antro-pyloro-duodenal motor response to gastric and duodenal nutrient in critically ill patients. Gut 2005;54:1384–1390.
23 Chapman MJ, Fraser RJ, Bryant LK, Vozzo R, Nguyen NQ, Tam W, Zacharakis B, Davidson G, Butler R, Horowitz M: Gastric emptying and the organization of antro-duodenal pressures in the critically ill. Neurogastroenterol Motil 2008;20:27–35.
24 Nguyen NQ, Fraser RJ, Brant LK, Chapman M, Holloway RH: Diminished functional association between proximal and distal gastric motility in critically ill patients. Intensive Care Med 2008;34:1246–1255.
25 Heyland DK, Tougas G, King D, et al: Impaired gastric emptying in mechanically ventilated, critically ill patients. Intensive Care Med 1996;22:1339–1344.
26 Kao CH, Chang Lai SP, Chieng PU, et al: Gastric emptying in head-injured patients. Am J Gastroenterol 1998;93:1108–1112.
27 Brand RE, DiBaise JK, Quigley EMM, et al: Gastroparesis as a cause of nausea and vomiting after high-dose chemotherapy and haemopoetic stem-cell transplantation. Lancet 1998;352:1985.

28 Deane AM, Dhaliwal R, Day AG, Ridley EJ, Davies AR, Heyland DK: Comparisons between intragastric and small intestinal delivery of enteral nutrition in the critically ill: a systematic review and meta-analysis. Crit Care 2013;17:R125.

29 Davies AR, Morrison SS, Bailey MJ, Bellomo R, Cooper DJ, Doig GS, Finfer SR, Heyland DK, ENTERIC Study Investigators, ANZICS Clinical Trials Group: A multicenter, randomized controlled trial comparing early nasojejunal with nasogastric nutrition in critical illness. Crit Care Med 2012;40:2342–2348.

30 Dall'Antonia M, Wilks M, Coen PG, Bragman S, Millar MR: Erythromycin for prokinesis: imprudent prescribing? Crit Care 2006;10:112.

31 Quigley EM: Passing the bug – translocation, bacteremia, and sepsis in the intensive care unit patient: is intestinal decontamination the answer? Crit Care Med 2011;39:1202–1203.

32 Fruhwald S, Kainz J: Effect of ICU interventions on gastrointestinal motility. Curr Op Crit Care 2010;16: 159–164.

33 Ponec RJ, Saunders MD, Kimmey MB: Neostigmine for the treatment of acute colonic pseudo-obstruction. New Eng J Med 1999;341:137–141.

34 Kayani B, Spalding DR, Jiao LR, Habib NA, Zacharakis E: Does neostigmine improve time to resolution of symptoms in acute colonic pseudo-obstruction? Int J Surg 2012;10:453–457.

35 Strodel WE, Brothers T: Colonoscopic decompression of pseudo-obstruction and volvulus. Surg Clin North Am 1989;69:1327–1335.

36 Eisner JL, Smith JM, Ensor CR: Intravenous neostigmine for post-operative acute colonic pseudo-obstruction. Ann Pharmacother 2012;46:430–435.

37 Rex DK: Colonoscopy and acute colonic pseudo-obstruction. Gastrointest Endosc Clin North Am 1997; 7:499–508.

38 Laine L: Management of acute colonic pseudo-obstruction. N Eng J Med 1999;341:192–193.

39 ASGE Standards of Practice Committee: The role of endoscopy in the management of patients with known and suspected colonic obstruction and pseudo-obstruction. Gastrointest Endosc 2010;71:669–679.

Eamonn M.M. Quigley, MD, FRCP, FACP, FACG, FRCPI
Division of Gastroenterology, The Methodist Hospital
6550 Fannin St, SM 2001
Houston, TX 77030 (USA)
E-Mail equigley@tmhs.org

Quigley EMM, Hongo M, Fukudo S (eds): Functional and GI Motility Disorders.
Front Gastrointest Res. Basel, Karger, 2014, vol 33, pp 141–149 (DOI: 10.1159/000356989)

Specific Clinical Contexts – Part 2: The Patient with Neurological Disease

Myung-Gyu Choi

Division of Gastroenterology, Department of Internal Medicine, College of Medicine, The Catholic University of Korea, Seoul, South Korea

Abstract

Gastrointestinal (GI) symptoms are common in patients with chronic neurological disease and have a major influence on quality of life, institutionalization rates and health care costs. However, GI symptoms are often underrecognized and poorly understood as clinicians focus mainly on severe motor disability or neurological deficits. The pathophysiology of GI symptoms in neurological disorders is likely to be multifactorial, involving abnormalities in reflexes and central pattern generators as well as autonomic outputs and enteric nerves. In some cases, the exact mechanisms leading to GI symptoms are still not understood completely. Parkinson's disease (PD) receives special attention because the pathophysiological abnormality involves the central, autonomic and enteric nervous systems. Furthermore, the early involvement of the GI tract in PD has important implications for our understanding of the pathophysiological and pathogenetic nature of PD, and might serve as an early biomarker to allow application of strategies intended to delay the onset of the motor symptoms. Further basic and clinical research aimed at elucidating the mechanisms underlying gut impairment in neurological disease is needed to develop diagnostic and therapeutic approaches for treating GI dysfunction.

Gastrointestinal (GI) symptoms are common in patients with chronic neurological disease and have a major influence on quality of life, institutionalization rates and health care costs. As the average age of our society increases, the prevalence of neurological diseases continues to increase and, therefore, consultations with gastroenterologists also increase [1]. The most common disorders that lead to consultations relating to GI motility problems are Parkinson's disease (PD) and cerebrovascular accidents, while the number of consultations because of Alzheimer's disease and other dementias may grow as the prevalence of these conditions increases. The prevalence of PD is estimated to be 0.3% in the general population and approximately 1% in people >60 years of age. In addition to its high prevalence, PD receives special attention because the pathophysiological abnormality involves the central, autonomic and enteric nervous systems (ENS). Recent studies have consistently indicated that ENS involvement occurs at an early stage of PD before brain lesions, supporting the hypothesis that the ENS may actually be the port of entry of the pathological process that eventually culminates in the clinical picture of PD.

Parkinson's Disease

Pathophysiology

PD is a multisystem disorder characterized by the involvement of selected neuronal populations throughout the central, autonomic and peripheral nervous systems. The pathological hallmark of PD, which causes the cardinal motor symptoms of tremor, rigidity and bradykinesia, is the degeneration of the dopaminergic melanized neurons of the substantia nigra pars compacta that project to the striatum. While PD has traditionally been considered a motor system disorder, it is now recognized to be a complex condition with diverse clinical features that include neuropsychiatric and other nonmotor manifestations, in addition to its motor symptomatology. GI symptoms, including excessive drooling, dysphagia, dyspepsia, nausea and constipation, are prominent nonmotor manifestations of PD [1–4]. GI symptoms occur not only in advanced PD, but also in its early stages, possibly more than a decade before the onset of motor symptoms [1, 3, 5, 6]. In a prospective observational study, 6,790 men without PD were tracked for 24 years, 1.4% of whom developed PD during the follow-up period. Interestingly, those patients with an initial finding of constipation were at threefold increased risk of developing PD after 10 years [5].

The neurodegeneration associated with PD is characterized by the formation of α-synuclein-containing inclusion bodies in the brain. Neuropathological studies show α-synuclein histopathology in the dorsal motor nucleus of the vagus (DMV) at the earliest stage of disease before the involvement of the substantia nigra [7–9]. The DMV provides parasympathetic innervation to much of the GI tract, so its involvement will play important roles in GI dysfunction. In PD, α-synuclein inclusions in the ENS, sympathetic and parasympathetic autonomic ganglia and DMV seem to follow a rostrocaudal gradient within the GI tract, being found most frequently in the submandibular gland and lower esophagus, followed by the stomach, small intestine, colon, and rectum [7, 10]. What is noteworthy is the extensive distribution of pathological α-synuclein inclusions in the ENS at the earliest stage of PD. Braak et al. [11] formulated the hypothesis that an exogenous pathogen might gain entry through peripheral nerve endings in the olfactory epithelium and GI mucosa, trigger local abnormal α-synuclein processing, and then pass from neuron to neuron in a prion-like fashion. The Braak model suggests that α-synuclein pathology starts in the gastric submucosal plexus and spreads to the central nervous system via axons of the DMV.

From the DMV, α-synuclein accumulation would spread to the midbrain and, finally, progress to the basal forebrain and neocortex [8, 10, 11]. This hypothesis is very intriguing as it suggests that environmental toxins or pathogens capable of passing the GI mucosal barrier may affect, in a retrograde fashion, α-synuclein processing in DMV neurons, leading to Lewy body pathology.

Experimental models provide further information about the potential neuropathological basis of GI dysfunction in PD [12]. Rats treated with rotenone develop myenteric α-synuclein aggregates similar to those observed in PD [13], and intragastric administration of a selective proteasome inhibitor in rats resulted in microglial activation and accumulation of intracytoplasmic α-synuclein inclusions in the DMV [14]. Early ENS involvement in PD could explain why objective parameters of GI dysmotility such as esophageal dysmotility, delayed gastric emptying and colonic transit are frequently observed in asymptomatic patients at an early stage of disease [1, 3, 15, 16]. Early involvement of the GI tract has important implications for our understanding of the pathophysiology and pathogenetics of PD, and might serve as an early biomarker to allow application of neuroprotective strategies intended to delay the onset of the motor symptoms of PD. Nonmotor features, including GI symptoms, could be used to detect and track PD.

GI symptoms could result from the motor symptoms of PD, which involve effects on the somatic innervation of the striated muscle components of the GI tract including the oropharynx, proximal esophagus, external anal sphincter, and pelvic floor muscles. Cognitive and neuropsychiatric symptoms ranging from anxiety, apathy and depression to dementia are frequently observed in patients with PD, and these may aggravate GI symptoms and impede their management. Medications used to treat the motor symptoms of PD, such as levodopa or anticholinergics, have been implicated in further slowing of GI motility and exacerbation of GI symptoms.

Oropharyngeal Dysphagia

The reported prevalence of dysphagia in patients with PD varies widely from 18.5 to 100% [4]. Progression of dysphagia leads to nutritional problems, poor quality of life and aspiration pneumonia, a common cause of death in patients with PD. Dysphagia typically occurs at late stages of the disease and correlates with motor disability. However, it is often unrecognized because many patients remain relatively asymptomatic even when abnormalities are demonstrated by video fluoroscopy and manometry [16–18]. All phases of swallowing can be impaired, with manifestations including poor bolus formation, lingual festination, and repetitive tongue elevation during the oral phase, delay of the swallow reflex, slowing of pharyngeal transit and pooling in the valleculae and pyriform sinuses during the pharyngeal phase and incomplete relaxation of the upper esophageal sphincter and abnormal esophageal peristalsis [19].

The determination of risk for aspiration is very important. Patients should be asked regularly if they have experienced any dysphagic symptoms and about recent weight loss or respiratory infections. However, subjective reports of swallowing function may not be accurate. This is of great concern because the risk of silent aspiration and resulting pneumonia may be present before the patient notices any overt symptoms of dysphagia. Objective evaluation of swallowing with video fluoroscopy is very sensitive and is used widely. It can accurately evaluate the oropharyngeal phase of swallowing, define dysfunction, and predict the therapeutic response. A recent elegant manometric study demonstrated that, not only a defective oropharyngeal phase of swallowing, but also esophageal dysmotility is present in a majority of newly diagnosed early-stage PD patients without severe motor symptoms, even before the clinical expression of dysphagia. Patients with PD often required multiple attempts to swallow a single bolus, and this was associated with abnormal peristalsis and incomplete transit. Abnormal responses were observed in the test of rapid multiple swallowing. This failed deglutitive inhibition reflects involvement of either the brainstem or the esophageal myenteric plexus [16]. These abnormal manometric findings may provide an early biomarker for the diagnosis of PD.

Optimal treatment of dysphagia involves a multidisciplinary approach in collaboration with a speech and language therapist. Gastroesophageal reflux disease could mimic or worsen dysphagia, and should be investigated and treated appropriately if found. Lifestyle modifications such as encouraging smaller bites at a slower rate, recommending thickening products and moist foods rather than thin liquids and eating in an upright chin-tuck position can be helpful. The benefits of treating dysphagia with antiparkinsonian medications are equivocal [4]. Although oral anticholinergic medications and antihistamines to reduce sialorrhea have been used clinically, their use should be reconsidered because drooling is not a result of excess salivation but rather reflect dysphagia. Botulinum toxin type A was reported in one clinical trial to be effective in reducing the frequency and severity of drooling [20].

Gastric Dysfunction

Delayed gastric emptying is reported in as many as 70–100% of PD patients [2, 3]. Gastroparesis can result in bothersome symptoms including nausea and vomiting, early satiety, and postprandial fullness. Delayed gastric emptying has been linked in some studies to the severity of motor impairment. However, a recent study showed delayed gastric emptying in 60% of PD patients at an early stage of disease [21]. The potential clinical relevance of delayed gastric emptying is that it could retard drug delivery and absorption, resulting in clinical fluctuations. *Helicobacter pylori* infection may contribute to GI symptoms and weight loss in PD. A recent trial demonstrated that *H. pylori* eradication improved the clinical status of infected patients with PD and reduced motor fluctuations, possibly by eliminating *H. pylori*-induced interference with L-dopa absorption [22]. These findings suggested the hypothesis that *Helicobacter* infection may play a causative role in the pathogenesis of PD by evoking autoimmunity against mitochondria, resulting in ENS damage [23].

Scintigraphy has been accepted as the gold standard test for measuring gastric emptying. In patients with neurological disease, the ^{13}C-octanoic acid breath test of gastric emptying has the advantage of simplicity and can be performed at the bedside in patients who are immobile or have dyskinetic movement [24]. The general management of symptomatic gastroparesis involves correcting fluid, electrolyte, and nutritional deficiencies, identifying and rectifying the underlying cause of gastroparesis, if possible, and reducing symptoms. Metoclopramide should be avoided in view of its central antidopaminergic effects. Domperidone is less likely to cross the blood-brain barrier and less likely to cause extrapyramidal side effects than metoclopramide. Mosapride is a 5-HT4 receptor agonist available in East Asia that accelerates gastric emptying. Erythromycin exerts strong prokinetic effects via action on motilin receptors. However, the lack of long-term efficacy of oral erythromycin and the possibility of the emergence of resistant bacterial strains limit its long-term use. For patients who are truly refractory to all pharmacotherapy, placement of a feeding jejunostomy and/or a venting gastrostomy can be considered. Use of total parenteral nutrition should be temporary, if possible, because of the risk of complications. Newer therapies currently being evaluated include intrapyloric injection of botulinum toxin and gastric electric stimulation, but their effectiveness in gastroparetic patients with PD is unclear.

Delayed Small and Large Bowel Transit and Anorectal Function

There is limited information on motility of the small intestine in PD. Acute and chronic intestinal pseudo-obstruction and megacolon have been reported in PD and other neurological diseases such as multiple sclerosis, motor neuron disease, Alzheimer's disease, autonomic neuropathies and in relation to spinal cord injury. Chronic megacolon may be asymptomatic depending on the level of consciousness and cognitive function and be discovered only on clinical or radiologic examination. Although the risk of perforation is apparently low, care should be taken as fatal outcomes have been reported [1]. Small intestinal bacterial overgrowth is highly prevalent in PD and is presumed to be a consequence of impaired motility of the small intestine [25]. In view of Braak's hypothesis, small intestinal bacterial overgrowth might not only represent a consequence of PD, but also play a role as an infectious agent that triggers the degenerative process in the ENS. This hypothesis should be tested further.

Constipation is a common nonmotor feature of PD and seems to be associated with PD severity. As mentioned above, constipation and slowed colonic transit may already be present in individuals with untreated early PD. Although slowed colonic transit is a major cause of constipation in PD, anorectal dysfunction, reduced tone of the diaphragm and abdominal muscles, drug therapy, poor oral intake and reduced physical activity also contribute to constipation. Anorectal dysfunction may be present in up to two thirds of individuals with PD [15]. It is influenced by the on and off stages, with improvement in the on stage and worsening in the off stage. Patients experiencing severe constipation refractory to pharmacologic intervention should be considered for anorectal function studies.

Colonic transit time can be measured noninvasively with the radio-opaque marker colonic transit test. Anorectal manometry can assess the integrity of the internal and external sphincters and is a well-established technique for the identification of anorectal dysfunction and incontinence. Manometry can be used as the basis for biofeedback approaches to improving sphincter function. Fluoroscopic defecography, anal sphincter electromyography and other tests can be utilized to evaluate anorectal function in PD patients. As PD patients usually have poor oral intake and decreased activity, encouraging fluid/fiber intake and physical activity are always recommended. Medication history should be reviewed and the anticholinergic burden assessed [20]. Laxatives are the backbone of constipation management. Several serotonin 5-HT4 receptor agonists have been evaluated in PD patients, and lubiprostone is currently being studied. Surgical treatment in the form of colectomy is necessary only in very rare instances in which megacolon or volvulus has developed. Biofeedback training has been studied or proven effective in treating anorectal dysfunction in some neurological disorders. The usefulness of biofeedback training has not been specifically evaluated in PD patients.

Cerebrovascular Accidents

After ischemic stroke, GI dysfunction can often be attributed directly to specific cerebral ischemic lesions involving the brain stem and certain cortical and subcortical structures. Dysphagia occurs in more than half of stroke patients immediately after the event and is a marker of poor prognosis, increasing the risks of pneumonia, malnutrition, persistent disability, prolonged hospital stay and mortality. Central control of swallowing involves both the brainstem and the cerebral cortex. While the reflexive component depends on swallowing centers in the brainstem, the initiation of swallowing is a voluntary action that involves multiple cortical regions, mainly within the sensorimotor cortex. The cortical representation of swallowing is thought to be multifocal and bilateral, with handedness-independent hemispheric dominance [26].

Dysphagia resolves spontaneously in most cortical stroke patients within 2 weeks of the onset of the stroke. However, the individual recovery pattern of patients who have similar severity of dysphagia at onset varies widely. The recovery of swallowing function relates to the reorganization of the remaining viable cerebral cortex and compensatory reorganization in functionally undamaged brain areas. This reorganization often occurs independently of the recovery of any associated hemiparesis and is not related to functional changes within the brainstem [26]. Therefore, interventions should not be hastily initiated, and patients should initially be assessed closely for aspiration risk and suitability for oral feeding. A variety of bedside assessments have been proposed that depend on the ability to swallow water or foods of various consistencies [27]. Bedside swallow tests are safe and therefore, repeatable and relatively straightforward to perform. However, many methods may miss silent aspiration, and assessments have reported a wide range of reliability. Although an abnormal gag reflex is associated with swallowing difficulties, in isolation it does not appear to predict aspiration risk. Video fluoroscopy and fiberoptic endoscopy may be useful but have their clinical limitations and should be interpreted with caution. Oxygen desaturation during swallowing may be predictive of aspiration but is more useful in combination with bedside testing than in isolation. Tube feeding may be an effective way of supplying nutrition in these patients, but its safety in terms of preventing aspiration is somewhat controversial. Like nasogastric tubes, gastrostomy tubes do not offer protection from colonization of oral secretions and are known to increase gastroesophageal reflux. A recent large trial suggests that nasogastric feeding should be used early for dysphagic patients, and percutaneous endoscopic gastrostomy feeding reserved for patients who do not tolerate nasogastric feeding and, possibly, as part of the long-term care of dysphagic patients [28]. Stimulation of the sensorimotor cortical representation of swallowing function using transcranial magnetic or direct current stimulation has promise as a method of inducing cortical plasticity after stroke, although its effect remains to be determined. Targeting the undamaged pharyngeal motor cortex has been reported to improve swallowing in healthy individuals and after dysphagic stroke [29].

Gastric emptying appears to be delayed following acute stroke and results in intolerance to enteral nutrition and unpredictable oral drug absorption. Stroke is also associated with constipation and anorectal dysfunction including incontinence, and instances of intestinal pseudo-obstruction have been reported. However, the pathophysiology of gastric, colonic and anorectal complications and complications of the small intestine in stroke patients are poorly understood. In most patients with ischemic stroke, colorectal dysfunction is caused by a combination of lesions of the central or peripheral nervous system, immobility, or altered dietary habits.

Alzheimer's Disease and Other Dementias

Adults older than 65 years demonstrate an increased prevalence of dementia estimated to be between 6 and 14%. The prevalence of dementia increases to over 30% beyond 85 years of age, and over 37% beyond 90 years. The number of GI consultations resulting from Alzheimer's disease and other dementias may grow as their prevalence increases. Dysphagia is a common symptom in dementia and has been reported in up to 45% of patients institutionalized with dementia. Dementia, dysphagia, and related feeding impairment can lead to nutritional deficits, which in turn contribute to pneumonia and mortality. Although little data have been published on the influence of Alzheimer's disease and other dementias on gastric, small-intestine and colorectal motility, GI dysfunction may be associated with malnutrition, weight loss and increased dependency, resulting in higher hospital admission rates and overall higher mortality.

Conclusions

GI symptoms in neurological disorders are often underrecognized and poorly understood as clinicians focus mainly on severe motor disability or neurological deficits. Motility tests can identify motor dysfunction as a cause of the patient's symptoms and are useful tools for investigating pathophysiological mechanisms. However, they are often not well tolerated because of motor disability and impaired cognitive function and therefore should be interpreted with caution. Management of GI symptoms is often very difficult because of comorbid neuropsychiatric conditions and concomitant drug therapy. Therefore, a normal finding in a global motility test is also clinically valuable to exclude severe GI dysmotility. The pathophysiology of GI symptoms in neurological disorders is likely to be multifactorial, involving abnormalities in reflexes and central pattern generators, as well as autonomic outputs and enteric nerves, and in some cases, the exact mechanisms leading to GI symptoms are not understood completely. Further basic and clinical research aimed at elucidating the mechanisms underlying gut impairment in neurological disease is needed to develop diagnostic and therapeutic approaches for treating GI dysfunction.

Acknowledgements

This study was supported in part by Business of Globalization for Science and Technology funded by the Ministry of Education, Science and Technology, Seoul, Republic of Korea (Grant NRF-2011-0031644).

References

1 Quigley EM, O'Mahony S, Heetun Z: Motility disorders in the patient with neurologic disease. Gastroenterol Clin North Am 2011;40:741–764.
2 Jost WH: Gastrointestinal dysfunction in Parkinson's disease. J Neurol Sci 2010;289:69–73.
3 Pfeiffer RF: Gastrointestinal dysfunction in Parkinson's disease. Parkinsonism Relat Disord 2011;17:10–15.
4 Wood LD, Neumiller JJ, Setter SM, Dobbins EK: Clinical review of treatment options for select nonmotor symptoms of Parkinson's disease. Am J Geriatr Pharmacother 2010;8:294–315.
5 Abbott RD, Petrovitch H, White LR, Masaki KH, Tanner CM, Curb JD, Grandinetti A, Blanchette PL, Popper JS, Ross GW: Frequency of bowel movements and the future risk of Parkinson's disease. Neurology 2001;57:456–462.
6 Krogh K, Ostergaard K, Sabroe S, Laurberg S: Clinical aspects of bowel symptoms in Parkinson's disease. Acta Neurol Scand 2008;117:60–64.
7 Beach TG, Adler CH, Sue LI, Vedders L, Lue L, White CL III, Akiyama H, Caviness JN, Shill HA, Sabbagh MN, Walker DG: Multi-organ distribution of phosphorylated alpha-synuclein histopathology in subjects with Lewy body disorders. Acta Neuropathol 2010;119:689–702.

8 Braak H, Del Tredici K, Rub U, de Vos RA, Jansen Steur EN, Braak E: Staging of brain pathology related to sporadic Parkinson's disease. Neurobiol Aging 2003;24:197–211.

9 Natale G, Pasquali L, Ruggieri S, Paparelli A, Fornai F: Parkinson's disease and the gut: a well known clinical association in need of an effective cure and explanation. Neurogastroenterol Motil 2008;20:741–749.

10 Cersosimo MG, Benarroch EE: Pathological correlates of gastrointestinal dysfunction in Parkinson's disease. Neurobiol Dis 2012;46:559–564.

11 Braak H, Rub U, Gai WP, Del Tredici K: Idiopathic Parkinson's disease: possible routes by which vulnerable neuronal types may be subject to neuroinvasion by an unknown pathogen. J Neural Transm 2003;110:517–536.

12 McDowell K, Chesselet MF: Animal models of the non-motor features of Parkinson's disease. Neurobiol Dis 2012;46:597–606.

13 Drolet RE, Cannon JR, Montero L, Greenamyre JT: Chronic rotenone exposure reproduces Parkinson's disease gastrointestinal neuropathology. Neurobiol Dis 2009;36:96–102.

14 Miwa H, Kubo T, Suzuki A, Kondo T: Intragastric proteasome inhibition induces alpha-synuclein-immunopositive aggregations in neurons in the dorsal motor nucleus of the vagus in rats. Neurosci Lett 2006;401:146–149.

15 Sung HY, Choi MG, Kim YI, Lee KS, Kim JS: Anorectal manometric dysfunctions in newly diagnosed, early-stage Parkinson's disease. J Clin Neurol 2012;8:184–189.

16 Sung HY, Kim JS, Lee KS, Kim YI, Song IU, Chung SW, Yang DW, Cho YK, Park JM, Lee IS, Kim SW, Chung IS, Choi MG: The prevalence and patterns of pharyngoesophageal dysmotility in patients with early stage Parkinson's disease. Mov Disord 2010;25:2361–2368.

17 Bushmann M, Dobmeyer SM, Leeker L, Perlmutter JS: Swallowing abnormalities and their response to treatment in Parkinson's disease. Neurology 1989;39:1309–1314.

18 Troche MS, Okun MS, Rosenbek JC, Musson N, Fernandez HH, Rodriguez R, Romrell J, Pitts T, Wheeler-Hegland KM, Sapienza CM: Aspiration and swallowing in Parkinson disease and rehabilitation with EMST: a randomized trial. Neurology 2010;75:1912–1919.

19 Ali GN, Wallace KL, Schwartz R, DeCarle DJ, Zagami AS, Cook IJ: Mechanisms of oral-pharyngeal dysphagia in patients with Parkinson's disease. Gastroenterology 1996;110:383–392.

20 Ondo WG, Hunter C, Moore W: A double-blind placebo-controlled trial of botulinum toxin B for sialorrhea in Parkinson's disease. Neurology 2004;62:37–40.

21 Krygowska-Wajs A, Cheshire WP Jr, Wszolek ZK, Hubalewska-Dydejczyk A, Jasinska-Myga B, Farrer MJ, Moskala M, Sowa-Staszczak A: Evaluation of gastric emptying in familial and sporadic Parkinson disease. Parkinsonism Relat Disord 2009;15:692–696.

22 Lee WY, Yoon WT, Shin HY, Jeon SH, Rhee PL: *Helicobacter pylori* infection and motor fluctuations in patients with Parkinson's disease. Mov Disord 2008;23:1696–1700.

23 Dobbs RJ, Dobbs SM, Weller C, Charlett A, Bjarnason IT, Curry A, Ellis DS, Ibrahim MA, McCrossan MV, O'Donohue J, Owen RJ, Oxlade NL, Price AB, Sanderson JD, Sudhanva M, Williams J: Helicobacter hypothesis for idiopathic parkinsonism: before and beyond. Helicobacter 2008;13:309–322.

24 Goetze O, Wieczorek J, Mueller T, Przuntek H, Schmidt WE, Woitalla D: Impaired gastric emptying of a solid test meal in patients with Parkinson's disease using 13C-sodium octanoate breath test. Neurosci Lett 2005;375:170–173.

25 Gabrielli M, Bonazzi P, Scarpellini E, Bendia E, Lauritano EC, Fasano A, Ceravolo MG, Capecci M, Rita Bentivoglio A, Provinciali L, Tonali PA, Gasbarrini A: Prevalence of small intestinal bacterial overgrowth in Parkinson's disease. Mov Disord 2011;26:889–892.

26 Schaller BJ, Graf R, Jacobs AH: Pathophysiological changes of the gastrointestinal tract in ischemic stroke. Am J Gastroenterol 2006;101:1655–1665.

27 Ramsey DJC, Smithard D, Kalra L: Early assessments of dysphagia and aspiration risk in acute stroke patients. Stroke 2003;34:1252–1257.

28 Dennis MS, Lewis SC, Warlow C: Effect of timing and method of enteral tube feeding for dysphagic stroke patients (FOOD): a multicentre randomised controlled trial. Lancet 2005;365:764–772.

29 Michou E, Mistry S, Jefferson S, Singh S, Rothwell J, Hamdy S: Targeting unlesioned pharyngeal motor cortex improves swallowing in healthy individuals and after dysphagic stroke. Gastroenterology 2012;142:29–38.

Prof. Myung-Gyu Choi
Division of Gastroenterology, Dept. of Internal Medicine, Seoul St. Mary's Hospital
The Catholic University of Korea, 505 Banpo-Dong
Seocho-Gu, 137-040 Seoul (South Korea)
E-Mail choim@catholic.ac.kr

Quigley EMM, Hongo M, Fukudo S (eds): Functional and GI Motility Disorders.
Front Gastrointest Res. Basel, Karger, 2014, vol 33, pp 150–162 (DOI: 10.1159/000356993)

Specific Clinical Contexts – Part 3: The Child with Neurodevelopmental Delay

Ryan Carvalho · Carlo Di Lorenzo

Division of Gastroenterology, Hepatology and Nutrition, Department of Pediatrics, Nationwide Children's Hospital, The Ohio State University Wexner College of Medicine, Columbus, Ohio, USA

Abstract

Varying degrees of gut dysmotility accompany the musculoskeletal disabilities of most children with neurodevelopmental delay. The majority of children with cerebral palsy, the most extensively studied among the diseases with neurodevelopmental delays, have clinically significant gastrointestinal symptoms, including swallowing difficulties, regurgitation and/or vomiting, pulmonary aspiration and chronic constipation. If inadequately diagnosed or treated, these disorders may result in malnutrition, growth delay and further impairment of the quality of life. Over the last two decades, considerable progress has been made in understanding the pathophysiologic mechanisms underlying gastrointestinal functional and motility disorders in pediatric patients. These findings have resulted in more specific diagnosis and the development of novel therapeutic approaches. Such advancement in neuroscience research has also helped gain considerable insight into the pathogenesis of symptoms in children with neurodevelopmental delay. This review focuses mostly on children with cerebral palsy and the clinical manifestations of their gastrointestinal motility dysfunctions. We describe the prevalence and clinical presentation of different disorders and discuss the diagnostic tests that have a role in their evaluation. Finally, we summarize the evidence supporting different medical and surgical treatment options.

Cerebral palsy (CP) also known as static encephalopathy represents a permanent, but not unchanging, disorder of movement or posture, and of motor function, caused by a non-progressive interference, lesion, or abnormality in the brain [1, 2]. Prematurity is a well-known risk factor for CP, and the risk of CP is inversely proportional to the gestational age of the premature infant. However, 50–65% of children with CP are born full term. Risk factors in term infants have been well defined in a recent systematic review and include placental abnormalities, birth defects, and neonatal infections among others [3].

The prevalence of CP over the previous two decades has been decreasing according to a multicenter European registry [4, 5]. However, this decrease in prevalence is not universal with certain centers reporting no difference and some even reporting increases in the prevalence of CP [6, 7]. While the musculoskeletal system is mainly affected, the pathogenesis of CP is primarily related to an injury of the central nervous system (CNS). Brain imaging studies in children with CP frequently show lesions involving the periventricular white matter and various patterns of dysgenesis and damage. These lesions are nonprogressive, but are responsible for the lack of normal neurophysiology in children with CP.

The nervous system exerts a profound influence on digestive processes, such as motility, ion transport, absorption, and gastrointestinal blood flow. Some of this control is derived from connections between the digestive tract and the CNS, in addition to interactions between the lumen and the enteric or intrinsic nervous system [8]. The myenteric plexus exerts control primarily over digestive tract motility. The submucous plexus plays a role in sensing the luminal environment, regulating gastrointestinal blood flow and controlling epithelial cell function. Normal digestive function requires sophisticated and functioning communication links between this intrinsic system and the CNS. These connections take the form of parasympathetic and sympathetic fibers that link either the central with the enteric nervous systems or allow the CNS to communicate directly with the digestive tract. Through these cross-connections, the gut can provide sensory afferent information to the CNS and the CNS can provide efferent regulation to the gastrointestinal function [9–12].

The link between the brain and enteric nervous system is becoming increasingly more understood. This crosstalk between what are considered the 'big brain' and the 'gut brain' is of great clinical significance since the degree of GI dysmotility seems to correlate with the degree of neurological damage to either system [13, 14]. Abnormalities in GI motility may sometimes be also an early presenting sign of underlying metabolic or mitochondrial disorders [15].

Modulation of the neural activity in the enteric nervous system by the extrinsic innervations is often abnormal in children with CNS disorders. Oral-motor skills parallel general neurological maturation [16]. Manometric studies in children with 'psychomotor retardation' have revealed incomplete relaxation of the upper esophageal sphincter and significantly decreased amplitude of peristaltic waves in the esophagus [13]. Gastrointestinal hormones and neuropeptides play an important role in the physiologic regulation of gastric emptying in children and in the transition from fasting to postprandial motility. Their role in causing motility dysfunction in children with neurodevelopmental abnormalities has not been determined yet but is speculated to be significant.

Gastroesophageal Reflux

The high incidence of gastroesophageal reflux (GER; 15–75%) in neurologically impaired children is well recognized [17–19]. Recurrent vomiting with aspiration and failure to thrive occurs in 10–15% of institutionalized children with psychomotor retardation related to disorders of the CNS [16]. Several hypotheses have been proposed to account for the high incidence of reflux in children with CP, including a high prevalence of hiatal hernias, prolonged supine position, abnormal muscle tone, obesity and increased intraabdominal pressure secondary to spasticity, scoliosis or seizures [20, 21].

In children with neurological impairment, the objective hallmark of GER disease (GERD) is recurrent vomiting which occurs in over 80% of cases and which may further compromise their already precarious nutritional state. Food-related behavior problems (food refusal, choking and coughing while eating, and poor weight gain) and rumination are common and found in about 40% of children with neurological impairment and GERD [22].

The association between GERD and respiratory complications (apnea, laryngitis, asthma/wheezing, chronic cough, chronic pulmonary aspiration, recurrent pneumonia, and progressive lung injury) has been recognized for decades [23].

An international consensus statement regarding the diagnosis of reflux in children and a clinical practice guideline on pediatric GER were published in 2009 [24, 25] and provide recommendations on how to approach children with or without neurodevelopmental delay in whom reflux is suspected. The evaluation of GERD in children with neurodevelopmental delays should be based on a high index of suspicion. Diagnostic studies which include contrast radiography, endoscopy with biopsy and intraesophageal pH monitoring/impedance often help to establish the diagnosis of reflux (table 1). Radiographic evaluation of the upper gastrointestinal tract is beneficial to uncover anatomical anomalies such as hiatal hernia, malrotation, antral or duodenal webs as well as previously unsuspected swallowed foreign bodies that could present with regurgitation and food refusal. Upper endoscopy shows different degrees of esophagitis in up to 80% of children who present with vomiting or regurgitation. It also helps to rule out other conditions such as eosinophilic esophagitis and infectious esophagitis, caused by candida and herpes viruses, and *Helicobacter pylori*-induced gastroduodenal mucosal disease. Intraesophageal pH studies typically show prolonged periods of acid exposure in the distal esophagus in children with neurodevelopmental delay and GERD. Simultaneous esophageal pH and impedance studies have demonstrated that a large number of nonacid reflux episodes can be missed by intraesophageal pH studies alone [26]. Using 12-hour impedance testing, Del Buono et al. [27] showed that in 16 neurologically impaired children more than half of the reflux events were nonacidic and would have gone undetected by conventional pH measurement.

The main esophageal motor abnormalities include low lower esophageal sphincter pressure, low amplitude esophageal body contractions and increased number of simultaneous, nonperistaltic waves [1]. Combined manometric and pH studies in the lower esophagus show that the associated esophageal dysmotility reduces the effectiveness of acid and pepsin clearance from the esophageal mucosa following GER episodes [13], increasing the risk for development of chronic esophagitis and Barrett's

Table 1. Indications, advantages and limitations of different diagnostic modalities to evaluate gastrointestinal motility

Test	Indications	Advantages	Limitations
Video fluoroscopic swallow study	choking and gagging with feeds, dysphagia, history of aspiration	widely available, tests for different food consistencies	radiation exposure, requires patient cooperation
Upper GI series	vomiting, chest pain, food refusal, dysphagia	widely available, detects anatomical abnormalities	radiation exposure, requires some patient cooperation
Esophageal pH-monitoring	atypical symptoms of reflux	widely available, normal values known	uncomfortable, 24-hour test
Esophageal impedance	atypical symptoms of reflux, before considering antireflux surgery	measures acid and non-acid reflux, correlates with atypical reflux symptoms	lack of reliable diagnostic standards for interpretation of results
Esophageal manometry	dysphagia, chest pain, suspicion of achalasia	direct measurement of motility	uncomfortable, not widely available
Upper endoscopy with biopsies	dysphagia, chronic reflux symptoms, vomiting, food impaction, chest pain	detects foregut mucosal lesions (esophagitis, gastritis duodenitis, celiac disease, infections, allergic diseases)	requires anesthesia, invasive, expensive
Gastric emptying scan	early satiety, bloating, vomiting, nausea	gold standard for diagnosis of gastroparesis	radiation exposure, long duration (4 h), not feasible if patient vomits test meal
Antroduodenal manometry	rumination, vomiting of unclear etiology	direct measure of fasting and postprandial foregut motility, correlation with symptoms	limited to few centers, requires sedation for probe placement, uncomfortable, long duration (6 h)
Sitz marker transit study	chronic constipation, concerns for colonic inertia	inexpensive, minimally invasive	radiation exposure
Colonic manometry	chronic constipation, concerns for colonic inertia	can test motility response to medications, identifies segmental defects	limited to few centers, requires anesthesia for probe placement, long duration (4 h)
Anorectal manometry	chronic constipation, Hirschsprung's disease, anal sphincter dysfunction, biofeedback treatment	easy to perform with cooperative patients	requires patient cooperation, difficult in younger patients, may require sedation

esophagus. Treatment of the esophagitis often improves esophageal motility [28]. Other explanations for the increased prevalence of reflux include the coexistence of gastric dysrhythmia, delayed gastric emptying and a low threshold for activation of the emetic reflex [16, 29, 30]. Indeed, two thirds of children with CP and GER had evidence of delayed gastric emptying [1]. Children with reflux at high risk for delayed gastric emptying include those with more severe neurologic disorders or brain damage, mental retardation, CP, Down syndrome (DS), and microcephaly. Because of the concern about gastroparesis, a gastric drainage procedure was performed at the same time as a fundoplication in 82% of children with CNS disorders compared to only 19% in those without CNS disorders in a large retrospective series [31]. The majority of patients with neurodevelopmental delay also required a feeding gastrostomy, and certain centers routinely perform an antireflux operation on almost all children with neurologic disorders at the time of the gastrostomy tube insertion. Antroduodenal motility studies in children with neurological impairment have revealed absent spontaneous fasting migrating motor complexes and postprandial hypomotility [32]. However, despite all currently available testing, a sizable number of patients with neurodevelopmental delay remain without a clear etiology for their recurrent vomiting.

Most patients with neurodevelopmental delay and GERD are primarily treated with acid suppression, with either an H2-blocker or a proton pump inhibitor (PPI). Vomiting usually persists despite acid suppression, although one small prospective study documented a reduction in emesis in neurologically impaired children treated with PPI [33]. Administration of baclofen has been shown to reduce the frequency of vomiting and the total number of acid reflux episodes in neurologically impaired children with GERD [34]. There is also some evidence that baclofen is beneficial in improving symptoms of GERD, and it accelerates gastric emptying [34, 35]. It is commonly observed that response to conventional medical therapy in this patient population is poor and antireflux surgery is frequently required. Irrespective of the surgical technique utilized, fundoplication is associated with higher morbidity and mortality rates in neurologically impaired children than in neurologically normal children [36–38]. Children with neurological impairment have a higher complication rate and an even higher rate of requiring reoperation [39]. In a study by Martinez et al. [37] more than a third of children with neurological impairment had major complications or died within 30 days of surgery and a quarter had documented operative failure. In some series, almost half of neurologically impaired children exhibited recurrent GER after surgery [36, 37]. Recurrent GER often leads to a second operation, but redo fundoplications fare no better with a failure rate of up to 28% noted in one study [40]. Retching and gas-bloat syndrome constitute frequent sequelae after fundoplication in children with neurological disability. Chronic, unremitting retching may have a dramatic impact on the quality of life of patients who have undergone a fundoplication and is seen more often in children with neurological disability than in normal children. Patients in whom retching already occurs preoperatively are three times more likely to retch following fundoplication than nonretchers [41, 42]. Administration of pureed food, fed through a gastrostomy has been shown to decrease gagging and retching behaviors in children after fundoplication [43]. However, in spite of these sequelae, a good number of caregivers report improved nutrition, decrease in reflux-related symptoms and high levels of satisfaction after fundoplication [44]. An alternative to antireflux surgery in children with severe GERD and vomiting is the creation of a feeding jejunostomy [45]. This surgery provides enteral access to maintain nutritional goals, while decreasing the risk of reflux and aspiration. However, it is limited by the requirement to administer nutrients only in a continuous fashion.

Initially described by Bianchi, the total esophagogastric disconnection represents a promising alternative approach to the feeding and vomiting problems that are so prevalent in children with neurodevelopmental delays. This surgery has proved successful even in children who have previously failed a fundoplication. The reoperation rate has been reported at 15%, and mortality rates vary between 11 and 28% [46–48]. Some authors are earnestly enthusiastic about this procedure and consider it to be the primary procedure for nutritional rehabilitation in neurologically impaired children [49].

Swallowing Difficulty

Even though tremendous progress has been made in the understanding of the normal swallow mechanism, a lot still remains unknown regarding the interaction between the hormonal and neuronal pathways involved in this complex physiological function. With a prevalence ranging from 40 to over 90%, dysphagia is relatively common in children with CP [50]. Food refusal is often a symptom related to various motor and sensory oropharyngeal disturbances in this patient population. In a large questionnaire survey, 20% of parents described feeding as stressful and unenjoyable [50]. Prolonged feeding times (>3 h per day) are a contributor to parental distress. In children with CP, oral-motor dysfunction is often the result of problems with the oral and the pharyngeal phases of swallowing [51]. Affected children were found to require more time than neurologically normal children for collection, preparation, oral transit, and total oral swallow time for liquid boluses. Total oral swallow time for solid bolus tasks was longer as well [52]. The majority of patients with CP and swallowing disorders demonstrate an abnormal formation of the food bolus and defective propulsion towards the pharynx. Less commonly but of more concern are disorders in the pharyngeal phase, often demonstrated by barium penetration and aspiration into the airway [53] (fig. 1).

If undiagnosed and untreated, complications of swallowing dysfunction include food refusal, aspiration, and recurrent pneumonia, which occur from 30 to over 70% depending on the neurological status of the patient and the study used to diagnose aspiration [54–56]. Aspiration may also be present without any of the typical symptoms of choking, gagging and coughing, a phenomenon called 'silent aspiration' [56]. However, aspiration could also be the consequence of moderate to severe GER [13, 14].

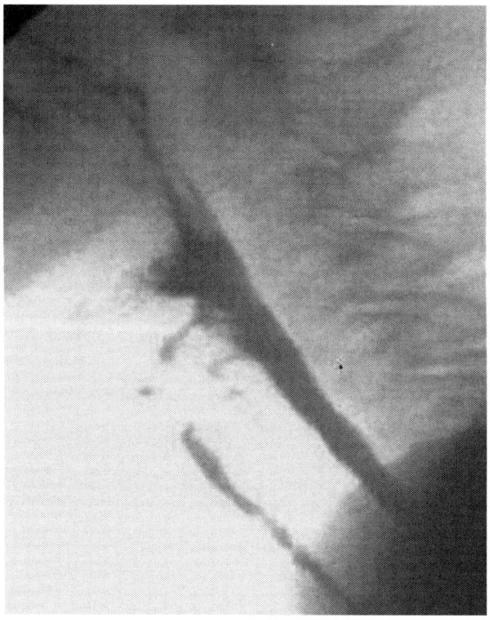

Fig. 1. Barium aspiration into the airway in a child undergoing a videoswallow study.

Severe swallow dysfunction with a risk of aspiration, nutritional compromise and reflux are common indications for placement of a percutaneous gastrostomy. There are well-described risks associated with gastrostomies in the neurologically compromised child. A number of case studies have reported that GER worsens when administering gastrostomy feeding [40, 57]. However, all these studies report an improvement in the nutritional status of these children. The majority of patients benefit from a multidisciplinary treatment which includes a variable combination of bolus or continuous pre- or postpyloric feedings, use of drugs to decrease visceral pain, medications for motility disorders, and behavioral, cognitive, and family therapy. The improved survival in children with severe neurological delays over the last two decades and the increased use of tube feeding to improve nutrition in this fragile population seem a likely association [58], although a systematic review to determine benefits and risks for gastrostomy or jejunostomy feedings compared to oral feedings for children with CP was inconclusive due to lack of high-quality evidence [59]. While there was a higher mortality reported in the gastrostomy group, these patients are often sicker, more severely impaired and with additional comorbidities.

Constipation

Constipation is a significant and common problem in neurologically impaired children and a manifestation of a probable underlying defect in gut innervations. Estimates of the prevalence of constipation vary from 26% to more than 50% of children with severe disabilities [60–62]. Abnormalities of colonic motility associated with neurological impairment include prolongation of colonic transit time in individuals with spinal cord injury [63] or meningomyelocele [64]. In a cross-sectional study of 38 children with spastic CP, all showed evidence of abnormal colonic transit time measured by the Metcalf criteria using radiopaque Sitz markers. A significant negative relationship between colon transit time and stool frequency was observed [62]. All neurodevelopmentally delayed children with constipation and even a majority without constipation showed an abnormal segmental colon transit time in at least one segment of the colon. A transit time delay at the proximal segment of colon was noted in many children with CP and constipation. In children without constipation, the transit time delay was more commonly appreciated in the rectosigmoid colon only, a common finding also in constipated children without neurologic impairment. Constipation and transit time delay were significantly related to ambulatory function with a longer transit time and more constipation in the nonambulators. A study using anorectal manometry in children with CP suggested that anal sphincter and/or pelvic floor muscle incoordination may also result in defecation difficulties [65].

Contributory factors to constipation include prolonged immobility, skeletal abnormalities, extensor spasm or generalized hypotonia, as well as abnormal bowel motility associated with certain neurological lesions [66–68]. Dietary factors such as low fiber intake and low fluid diets (often due to associated feeding difficulties) represent important contributors as well. Constipation has also been reported to be a fairly common complication of a ketogenic diet, which is often used to treat refractory epilepsy in many children with a variety of congenital or acquired neurological diseases [69]. The use of anticonvulsant, opioid, antispasmodic, antihistamine, or aluminum antacid medications in disabled children may also predispose to constipation.

Constipation in these children presents with large hard stools, infrequent bowel movements and pain or irritability with defecation. Chronic constipation has been associated with impaired quality of life, increased prevalence of urinary symptoms (e.g. dysfunctional voiding, recurrent urinary tract infection, and deterioration of vesicoureteric reflux) as well as other gastrointestinal symptoms (e.g. recurrent vomiting, early satiety, poor feeding, chronic nausea and chronic or recurrent abdominal pain).

Children with neurodisabilities often have lower intake of fiber and water [60]. While fiber supplementation has not been universally successful in the treatment of constipation, some small studies in nonambulatory enterally fed children with varying degrees of neurological impairment have shown that adding soy-polysaccharide fiber at doses between 18–25 g per day significantly increased mean daily stool frequency. Lower doses of 12–20 g per day significantly increased stool moisture and wet stool weight [70]. Use of glucomannan (a water soluble polysaccharide) also led to a significantly increased stool frequency. Its use was associated with a reduction in other laxative or suppository use, and stool consistency and episodes of painful defecation improved as well [71]. However, neither glucomannan nor fiber had a measurable effect on total and segmental transit times.

The use of preparations containing mineral oil should be avoided in children with concomitant neurological abnormalities and GER due to the increased risk of aspiration [72]. Though largely removed from the US market, cisapride is still used in some countries and can be accessed on a compassionate basis in the US. However, the evidence for recommending this prokinetic in children with constipation with neurological deficit is modest at best. A single-center, double-blind trial showed an improvement in stool frequency, but the improvement was similar in the control group. Although cisapride helped to significantly reduce the use of laxatives or suppositories, it had no effect on total gastrointestinal transit time and colonic segmental transit time [73].

Once medical, dietary and behavioral treatments have failed to improve the defecatory problem, surgical options are often entertained. The antegrade continence enema procedure has been reported to have an 80% success rate. Best results are achieved in children greater than 5 years old with a neuropathic bowel or anorectal malformations who are highly motivated to remain continent [74]. A retrospective review looking at 10 years of experience using antegrade enemas as a treatment strategy for children with chronic constipation included 9 children with CP. The majority of the children improved and a few children, including one with CP, were able to successfully discontinue the use of antegrade enemas and remain symptom free after 24 months. This procedure warrants further study in this patient population [75].

Other Conditions

Special categories include children with DS and Rett syndrome (RS). While the variation in the phenotype of these conditions is considerable, children with DS are considered to be at an increased risk for GERD, achalasia, feeding difficulties, chronic constipation and Hirschsprung's disease [14, 76, 77]. They also seem to have more complications of reflux such as aspiration and pneumonia [78]. Studies have attributed these events to a lack of self-protective mechanisms in addition to impaired esophageal clearance, abnormal swallowing, delayed gastric emptying and abnormal muscle tone [79]. Achalasia also has a higher prevalence in children with DS and must be considered in the differential diagnosis for children presenting with chronic regurgitation and worsening vomiting [80]. Much like children with CP, children with DS often require surgery to improve refractory GERD.

Girls with RS have a high prevalence of feeding difficulties (81%), GER (39%), and constipation (80%) [81, 82]. Feeding problems were more specifically noted to be associated with chewing difficulty, prolonged feeding time, swallowing abnormalities and choking/gagging with feedings. Most girls with RS displayed one or more features of gastroesophageal dysmotility by radiographic criteria. Esophageal and gastric dysmotility is present in nearly half of them. An important finding was the relatively high rate of Barrett's esophagitis, emphasizing the need for endoscopic screening in this patient population. Interestingly, subjects with an MECP2 mutation were less likely to have chewing difficulty, choking or gagging with feeding, or night-time awakening with irritability than those without an MECP2 mutation. Vomiting or regurgitation, night-time awakening with irritability, GER, chewing difficulty, and choking or gagging with feeding were more likely to occur in younger (less than 14 years of age) individuals [81, 82].

For children with neurodevelopmental disability, active engagement with a multidisciplinary team including pediatricians, gastroenterologists, ear-nose-throat specialists, pulmonologists, speech pathologists, rehabilitation experts, neurologists, nurses, and nutritionists represents the most effective way to improve their quality of life.

References

1 Del Giudice E, Staiano A, Capano G, et al: Gastrointestinal manifestations in children with cerebral palsy. Brain Dev 1999;21:307–311.
2 Allen MC: Neurodevelopmental outcomes of preterm infants. Curr Opin Neurol 2008;21:123–128.
3 McIntyre S, Taitz D, Keogh J, et al: A systematic review of risk factors for cerebral palsy in children born at term in developed countries. Dev Med Child Neurol 2013;55:499–508.
4 Andersen GL, Romundstad P, De La Cruz J, et al: Cerebral palsy among children born moderately preterm or at moderately low birthweight between 1980 and 1998: a European register-based study. Dev Med Child Neurol 2011;53:913–919.
5 Platt MJ, Cans C, Johnson A, et al: Trends in cerebral palsy among infants of very low birthweight (<1,500 g) or born prematurely (<32 weeks) in 16 European centres: a database study. Lancet 2007;369:43–50.
6 Hoon AH Jr: Neuroimaging in cerebral palsy: patterns of brain dysgenesis and injury. J Child Neurol 2005;20:936–939.
7 Winter S, Autry A, Boyle C, Yeargin-Allsopp M: Trends in the prevalence of cerebral palsy in a population-based study. Pediatrics 2002;110:1220–1225.
8 Goyal RK, Hirano I: The enteric nervous system. N Engl J Med 1996;334:1106–1115.
9 Furness JB, Costa M: Types of nerves in the enteric nervous system. Neuroscience 1980;5:1–20.
10 Gershon MD, Kirchgessner AL, Wade PR (ed): Functional anatomy of the enteric nervous system; in Johnson LR, Alpers DH, Jacobson ED, Walsh JH (eds): Physiology of the Gastrointestinal Tract. New York, Raven Press, 1994, pp 381–422.
11 Costa M, Brookes SJ: The enteric nervous system. Am J Gastroenterol 1994;89(suppl 8):S129–S137.
12 Furness JB, Bernstein JC, Kunze WA, Clerc N: The enteric nervous system and its extrinsic connections; in Yamada T (ed): Textbook of Gastroenterology, ed 2. Philadelphia, Lippincott Williams & Wilkins, 1995, vol 1, pp 2–24.
13 Staiano A, Cucchiara S, Del Giudice E, et al: Disorders of oesophageal motility in children with psychomotor retardation and gastro-oesophageal reflux. Eur J Pediatr 1991;150:638–641.
14 Martinelli M, Staiano A: Motility problems in the intellectually challenged child, adolescent, and young adult. Gastroenterol Clin North Am 2011;40:765–775, viii.
15 Chitkara DK, Nurko S, Shoffner JM, et al: Abnormalities in gastrointestinal motility are associated with diseases of oxidative phosphorylation in children. Am J Gastroenterol 2003;98:871–877.
16 Ravelli AM, Milla PJ: Vomiting and gastroesophageal motor activity in children with disorders of the central nervous system. J Pediatr Gastroenterol Nutr 1998;26:56–63.
17 Gustafsson PM, Tibbling L: Gastro-oesophageal reflux and oesophageal dysfunction in children and adolescents with brain damage. Acta Paediatr 1994; 83:1081–1085.
18 Wesley JR, Coran AG, Sarahan TM, et al: The need for evaluation of gastroesophageal reflux in brain-damaged children referred for feeding gastrostomy. J Pediatr Surg 1981;16:866–871.

19 Reyes AL, Cash AJ, Green SH, Booth IW: Gastrooesophageal reflux in children with cerebral palsy. Child Care Health Dev 1993;19:109–118.
20 Halpern LM, Jolley SG, Johnson DG: Gastroesophageal reflux: a significant association with central nervous system disease in children. J Pediatr Surg 1991;26:171–173.
21 Harrington JW, Brand DA, Edwards KS: Seizure disorder as a risk factor for gastroesophageal reflux in children with neurodevelopmental disabilities. Clin Pediatr (Phila) 2004;43:557–562.
22 Bohmer CJ, Klinkenberg-Knol EC, Niezen-de Boer MC, Meuwissen SG: Gastroesophageal reflux disease in intellectually disabled individuals: how often, how serious, how manageable? Am J Gastroenterol 2000;95:1868–1872.
23 Orenstein SR, Orenstein DM: Gastroesophageal reflux and respiratory disease in children. J Pediatr 1988;112:847–858.
24 Sherman PM, Hassall E, Fagundes-Neto U, et al: A global, evidence-based consensus on the definition of gastroesophageal reflux disease in the pediatric population. Am J Gastroenterol 2009;104:1278–1295, quiz 1296.
25 Vandenplas Y, Rudolph CD, Di Lorenzo C, et al: Pediatric gastroesophageal reflux clinical practice guidelines: joint recommendations of the North American Society for Pediatric Gastroenterology, Hepatology, and Nutrition (NASPGHAN) and the European Society for Pediatric Gastroenterology, Hepatology, and Nutrition (ESPGHAN). J Pediatr Gastroenterol Nutr 2009;49:498–547.
26 Wenzl TG: Evaluation of gastroesophageal reflux events in children using multichannel intraluminal electrical impedance. Am J Med 2003;115(suppl 3A):161S–165S.
27 Del Buono R, Wenzl TG, Rawat D, Thomson M: Acid and nonacid gastro-oesophageal reflux in neurologically impaired children: investigation with the multiple intraluminal impedance procedure. J Pediatr Gastroenterol Nutr 2006;43:331–335.
28 Cucchiara S, Staiano A, Di Lorenzo C, et al: Esophageal motor abnormalities in children with gastroesophageal reflux and peptic esophagitis. J Pediatr 1986;108:907–910.
29 Andrews PL, Hawthorn J: The neurophysiology of vomiting. Baillieres Clin Gastroenterol 1988;2:141–168.
30 Andrews PL, Richards CA, Smith JE: The neurophysiology of emesis: lessons from basic science for understanding paediatric problems. J Pediatr Gastroenterol Nutr 2001;32(suppl 1):S12–S13.
31 Fonkalsrud EW, Ament ME, Vargas J: Gastric antroplasty for the treatment of delayed gastric emptying and gastroesophageal reflux in children. Am J Surg 1992;164:327–331.
32 Werlin SL: Antroduodenal motility in neurologically handicapped children with feeding intolerance. BMC Gastroenterol 2004;4:19.
33 Cheung KM, Tse PW, Ko CH, et al: Clinical efficacy of proton pump inhibitor therapy in neurologically impaired children with gastroesophageal reflux: prospective study. Hong Kong Med J 2001;7:356–359.
34 Kawai M, Kawahara H, Hirayama S, et al: Effect of baclofen on emesis and 24-hour esophageal pH in neurologically impaired children with gastroesophageal reflux disease. J Pediatr Gastroenterol Nutr 2004;38:317–323.
35 Omari TI, Benninga MA, Sansom L, et al: Effect of baclofen on esophagogastric motility and gastroesophageal reflux in children with gastroesophageal reflux disease: a randomized controlled trial. J Pediatr 2006;149:468–474.
36 Martinez DA, Ginn-Pease ME, Caniano DA: Recognition of recurrent gastroesophageal reflux following antireflux surgery in the neurologically disabled child: high index of suspicion and definitive evaluation. J Pediatr Surg 1992;27:983–988, discussion 988–990.
37 Martinez DA, Ginn-Pease ME, Caniano DA: Sequelae of antireflux surgery in profoundly disabled children. J Pediatr Surg 1992;27:267–271, discussion 271–273.
38 Esposito C, Van Der Zee DC, Settimi A, et al: Risks and benefits of surgical management of gastroesophageal reflux in neurologically impaired children. Surg Endosc 2003;17:708–710.
39 Pearl RH, Robie DK, Ein SH, et al: Complications of gastroesophageal antireflux surgery in neurologically impaired versus neurologically normal children. J Pediatr Surg 1990;25:1169–1173.
40 Subramaniam R, Dickson AP: Long-term outcome of Boix-Ochoa and Nissen fundoplication in normal and neurologically impaired children. J Pediatr Surg 2000;35:1214–1216.
41 Richards CA, Andrews PL, Spitz L, Milla PJ: Nissen fundoplication may induce gastric myoelectrical disturbance in children. J Pediatr Surg 1998;33:1801–1805.
42 Richards CA, Milla PJ, Andrews PL, Spitz L: Retching and vomiting in neurologically impaired children after fundoplication: predictive preoperative factors. J Pediatr Surg 2001;36:1401–1404.
43 Pentiuk S, O'Flaherty T, Santoro K, et al: Pureed by gastrostomy tube diet improves gagging and retching in children with fundoplication. JPEN J Parenter Enteral Nutr 2011;35:375–379.
44 O'Loughlin EV, Somerville H, Shun A, et al: Antireflux surgery in children with neurological impairment: caregiver perceptions and complications. J Pediatr Gastroenterol Nutr 2013;56:46–50.

45 Esposito C, Settimi A, Centonze A, et al: Laparoscopic-assisted jejunostomy: an effective procedure for the treatment of neurologically impaired children with feeding problems and gastroesophageal reflux. Surg Endosc 2005;19:501–504.
46 Danielson PD, Emmens RW: Esophagogastric disconnection for gastroesophageal reflux in children with severe neurological impairment. J Pediatr Surg 1999;34:84–86, discussion 87.
47 Bianchi A: Total esophagogastric dissociation: an alternative approach. J Pediatr Surg 1997;32:1291–1294.
48 Buratti S, Kamenwa R, Dohil R, et al: Esophagogastric disconnection following failed fundoplication for the treatment of gastroesophageal reflux disease (GERD) in children with severe neurological impairment. Pediatr Surg Int 2004;20:786–790.
49 Gatti C, di Abriola GF, Villa M, et al: Esophagogastric dissociation versus fundoplication: which is best for severely neurologically impaired children? J Pediatr Surg 2001;36:677–680.
50 Parkes J, Hill N, Platt MJ, Donnelly C: Oromotor dysfunction and communication impairments in children with cerebral palsy: a register study. Dev Med Child Neurol 2010;52:1113–1119.
51 Casas MJ, Kenny DJ, McPherson KA: Swallowing/ventilation interactions during oral swallow in normal children and children with cerebral palsy. Dysphagia 1994;9:40–46.
52 Casas MJ, McPherson KA, Kenny DJ: Durational aspects of oral swallow in neurologically normal children and children with cerebral palsy: an ultrasound investigation. Dysphagia 1995;10:155–159.
53 Zangen T, Ciarla C, Zangen S, et al: Gastrointestinal motility and sensory abnormalities may contribute to food refusal in medically fragile toddlers. J Pediatr Gastroenterol Nutr 2003;37:287–293.
54 Mirrett PL, Riski JE, Glascott J, Johnson V: Videofluoroscopic assessment of dysphagia in children with severe spastic cerebral palsy. Dysphagia 1994;9:174–179.
55 Rogers B, Arvedson J, Buck G, et al: Characteristics of dysphagia in children with cerebral palsy. Dysphagia 1994;9:69–73.
56 Arvedson J, Rogers B, Buck G, et al: Silent aspiration prominent in children with dysphagia. Int J Pediatr Otorhinolaryngol 1994;28:173–181.
57 Heine RG, Reddihough DS, Catto-Smith AG: Gastro-oesophageal reflux and feeding problems after gastrostomy in children with severe neurological impairment. Dev Med Child Neurol 1995;37:320–329.
58 Strauss D, Shavelle R, Reynolds R, et al: Survival in cerebral palsy in the last 20 years: signs of improvement? Dev Med Child Neurol 2007;49:86–92.
59 Sleigh G, Brocklehurst P: Gastrostomy feeding in cerebral palsy: a systematic review. Arch Dis Child 2004;89:534–539.
60 Veugelers R, Benninga MA, Calis EA, et al: Prevalence and clinical presentation of constipation in children with severe generalized cerebral palsy. Dev Med Child Neurol 2010;52:e216–e221.
61 Tse PW, Leung SS, Chan T, et al: Dietary fibre intake and constipation in children with severe developmental disabilities. J Paediatr Child Health 2000;36:236–239.
62 Elawad MA, Sullivan PB: Management of constipation in children with disabilities. Dev Med Child Neurol 2001;43:829–832.
63 Keshavarzian A, Barnes WE, Bruninga K, et al: Delayed colonic transit in spinal cord-injured patients measured by indium-111 Amberlite scintigraphy. Am J Gastroenterol 1995;90:1295–1300.
64 Pigeon N, Leroi AM, Devroede G, et al: Colonic transit time in patients with myelomeningocele. Neurogastroenterol Motil 1997;9:63–70.
65 Agnarsson U, Warde C, McCarthy G, et al: Anorectal function of children with neurological problems. II. cerebral palsy. Dev Med Child Neurol 1993;35:903–908.
66 Weber J, Denis P, Mihout B, et al: Effect of brainstem lesion on colonic and anorectal motility. Study of three patients. Dig Dis Sci 1985;30:419–425.
67 Staiano A, Del Giudice E: Colonic transit and anorectal manometry in children with severe brain damage. Pediatrics 1994;94:169–173.
68 Park ES, Park CI, Cho SR, et al: Colonic transit time and constipation in children with spastic cerebral palsy. Arch Phys Med Rehabil 2004;85:453–456.
69 Mackay MT, Bicknell-Royle J, Nation J, et al: The ketogenic diet in refractory childhood epilepsy. J Paediatr Child Health 2005;41:353–357.
70 Liebl BH, Fischer MH, Van Calcar SC, Marlett JA: Dietary fiber and long-term large bowel response in enterally nourished nonambulatory profoundly retarded youth. JPEN J Parenter Enteral Nutr 1990;14:371–375.
71 Staiano A, Simeone D, Del Giudice E, et al: Effect of the dietary fiber glucomannan on chronic constipation in neurologically impaired children. J Pediatr 2000;136:41–45.
72 Bandla HP, Davis SH, Hopkins NE: Lipoid pneumonia: a silent complication of mineral oil aspiration. Pediatrics 1999;103:E19.
73 Staiano A, Del Giudice E, Simeone D, et al: Cisapride in neurologically impaired children with chronic constipation. Dig Dis Sci 1996;41:870–874.
74 Malone PS: The antegrade continence enema procedure. BJU Int 2004;93:248–249.
75 Mugie SM, Machado RS, Mousa HM, et al: Ten-year experience using antegrade enemas in children. J Pediatr 2012;161:700–704.

76 van Trotsenburg AS, Heymans HS, Tijssen JG, et al: Comorbidity, hospitalization, and medication use and their influence on mental and motor development of young infants with Down syndrome. Pediatrics 2006;118:1633–1639.
77 Moore SW: Down syndrome and the enteric nervous system. Pediatr Surg Int 2008;24:873–883.
78 Seki M, Kato T, Masutani S, et al: Pulmonary arterial hypertension associated with gastroesophageal reflux in a 2-month-old boy with Down syndrome. Circ J 2009;73:2352–2354.
79 Hillemeier C, Buchin PJ, Gryboski J: Esophageal dysfunction in Down's syndrome. J Pediatr Gastroenterol Nutr 1982;1:101–104.
80 Zarate N, Mearin F, Gil-Vernet JM, et al: Achalasia and Down's syndrome: coincidental association or something else? Am J Gastroenterol 1999;94:1674–1677.
81 Motil KJ, Schultz RJ, Browning K, et al: Oropharyngeal dysfunction and gastroesophageal dysmotility are present in girls and women with Rett syndrome. J Pediatr Gastroenterol Nutr 1999;29:31–37.
82 Motil KJ, Caeg E, Barrish JO, et al: Gastrointestinal and nutritional problems occur frequently throughout life in girls and women with Rett syndrome. J Pediatr Gastroenterol Nutr 2012;55:292–298.

Carlo Di Lorenzo, MD
The Ohio State Univ. Wexner College of Medicine, Division of Gastroenterology
Nationwide Children's Hospital, 700 Children's drive
Columbus, OH 43205 (USA)
E-Mail Carlo.DiLorenzo@nationwidechildrens.org

Quigley EMM, Hongo M, Fukudo S (eds): Functional and GI Motility Disorders.
Front Gastrointest Res. Basel, Karger, 2014, vol 33, pp 163–169 (DOI: 10.1159/000356997)

Specific Clinical Contexts – Part 4: The Postoperative Patient

Gabrio Bassotti[a] · Vincenzo Villanacci[b] · Edda Battaglia[c] · Christoph Andreas Maurer[d]

[a]Gastroenterology and Hepatology Section, Department of Clinical and Experimental Medicine, University of Perugia, Perugia, [b]Second Pathology Section, Spedali Civili, Brescia, and [c]Gastroenterology Unit, Cardinal Massaja Hospital, Asti, Italy; [d]Department of Surgery, Hospital of Baselland affiliated with the University of Basel, Liestal, Switzerland

Abstract

All surgical procedures on the gastrointestinal tract may influence the homeostasis of gut motility, and often the surgical results are intimately linked to the onset of motor disturbances. Depending on the surgical approach, these postoperative dysmotilities may influence to a lesser or greater extent the quality of life of patients undergoing surgery of the gastrointestinal tract. This chapter will briefly review some concepts related to these motor abnormalities that can follow gut surgery.

Surgical interventions on the gastrointestinal tract may all, to a greater or lesser extent, influence gut motility. This may happen chiefly through resections that remove minor or major portions of the hollow viscera, although other albeit less invasive procedures (such as myotomies) may also play an important role in causing postoperative gut dysmotility.

Thus, upper gut surgical procedures will influence the normal motor function of the esophagus, mainly devoted to the transport of the ingesta from the mouth to the stomach, of the stomach, altering gastric emptying, and of the small bowel, disturbing the motor homeostasis that allows optimal absorption and clearance of the ingested substances [1].

Minor or major surgical resections involving the colorectal area will disrupt normal motor function, with disorganization of both the basal (segmental) activity at rest and after eating, and the propagated activity that leads to defecation; the latter consists of a sequence of well-integrated motor events starting from the terminal ileum and – through coordination with colorectal and anal structures – culminating with the expulsion of stools and/or flatus [2, 3].

Postoperative influences on gut motility may be acute and transient (postoperative ileus) or may become a chronic, persistent state due to the need to adapt to a new anatomic and physiologic condition.

Postoperative Ileus

This term defines a clinical condition that occurs in almost all patients undergoing major gut surgery, and is characterized by abdominal distension, nausea, vomiting, and inability to defecate or tolerate a solid diet [4]. Postoperative ileus is secondary to a transient interruption of bowel function with a variable reduction in motility sufficient to prevent effective transit of intestinal contents [4]. The pathophysiologic basis of postoperative ileus rests on at least three (often intermeshing) mechanisms, summarized as follows [5]: (1) Neurogenic inhibition of the bowel, related to a pain-induced neural reflex, causing sympathetic hyperactivity and release of endogenous opioids, with subsequent reduction (up to absence) of gastrointestinal motility. (2) Inhibition of gastrointestinal smooth muscle, due to localized postoperative inflammation. There is recent evidence that intestinal inflammation, triggered by handling of the bowel, represents one of the main mechanisms leading to ileus development, by activation of quiescent mast cells and macrophages that release inflammatory substances able to inhibit gut motility via inflammatory cascades mediated through the arachidonic acid pathway [6]. (3) Inhibition of bowel motility secondary to the use of opioids, compounds that reduce gastrointestinal secretion and inhibit the contractile activity of the gut.

Esophageal Surgery

The motor function of the esophagus may be affected by several surgical procedures carried out for neoplastic (i.e. adenocarcinoma or squamous cell carcinoma) or benign (i.e. achalasia, gastroesophageal reflux disease, GERD) conditions that can (and often will) influence peristalsis and anti-reflux mechanisms.

Achalasia

The three traditional treatment options for achalasia are surgical myotomy, pneumatic dilation, and botulinum toxin injection. Botulinum is a safe and easy treatment choice when surgical intervention is considered high risk, and with good results especially in older patients [7]. The surgical approach usually consists of an esophageal myotomy often with a partial fundoplication, with a success rate >90%. With the development of minimally invasive techniques, the surgical approach, and particularly the laparoscopic one, has gained widespread acceptance among patients and gastroenterologists, even though follow-up studies have not shown a superior therapeutic gain compared to pneumatic dilatation [8]. It is worth noting that, despite the symptom improvement offered to achalasia patients by either pneumatic dilation or surgical myotomy, 10–15% of those so treated will present with progressive deterioration of their esophageal function, and up to 5% may eventually require an esophagectomy [9]. Limited distal esophagectomy with short-colon interposition through a left thoracoabdominal approach is a safe and feasible alternative to near-total esophagectomy in patients with achalasia who have failed esophagomyotomy, offering an improvement in alimentary function and a better quality of life after the operation [10].

Gastroesophageal Reflux Disease

Surgical treatment for GERD is reserved for selected patients, affected by severe forms of the disease, or refractory to treatment, and/or noncompliance to medical therapy. A notable improvement of the quality of life is observed in up to 80% of patients submitted to antireflux surgery [11], and the Nissen-Rossetti minimally invasive approach is performed with acceptable complication rates (3–10%) [12]. The most frequent complication of fundoplication is dysphagia. Although, historically, this symptom has been related to preoperative esophageal body motility, this has proven to be an unreliable predictor of postoperative dysphagia. Recent data suggest that postoperative alterations in hiatal functional anatomy, such as impaired relaxation of the neo-high pressure zone, are the primary factors responsible for post-Nissen dysphagia [13]. It remains to be established whether high-resolution manometry will prove more useful in revealing esophageal motor disorders associated with dysphagia and also in demonstrating, preoperatively, esophageal motor function abnormalities that are more predictive of a poor postoperative outcome or, on the contrary, more severe GERD [14].

Esophageal Cancer

Esophagectomy via a cervico-thoraco-abdominal approach is a useful surgical technique to treat patients with esophageal cancer. Reconstruction with various components of the gastrointestinal tract (stomach, colon or small bowel), however, is associated with a high rate of anastomotic leakage, as well as anastomotic stricture, intrathoracic stomach syndrome, reflux esophagitis and other complications, thereby influencing postoperative recovery and quality of life. Short- and long-term functional outcomes are affected by the type of reconstruction performed after esophagectomy, with dysphagia and heartburn being the main postoperative symptoms. Esophageal replacement with a gastric tube is a well-established mode of reconstruction after esophagectomy in cancer patients, but severe hypoperistalsis in the residual esophagus and absent motor activity in the gastric tube, leading to pathological levels of esophageal acid exposure, may result. Hypomotility of the residual esophagus and gastric tube seems to be closely associated with disruption of the SCF/c-kit signaling pathway [15].

Gastric and Intestinal Surgery

It is now well known that almost any surgical procedure on the stomach and small bowel may, to a greater or lesser extent, influence the motor activity of the residual bowel. However, specific studies on this topic are relatively few [16, 17]. The formation of a pouch reservoir as a gastric substitute has repeatedly been advocated to be clinically advantageous and to improve quality of life after total gastrectomy. However, available data have not shown convincingly that pouch reconstruction is the technique of choice [18]. Concerning reconstruction after distal gastrectomy for gastric cancer, duodenal-esophageal reflux after a Roux-en-Y anastomosis procedure is significantly less frequent than after other types of anastomoses, such as Billroth I or Billroth II with Braun anastomosis, despite the fact that there is no difference in the postoperative quality of life index and nutritional status between the various reconstructive procedures [19].

Owing to the fact that obesity had become a major medical problem worldwide, bariatric surgery has greatly expanded in recent years. Even though several therapeutic approaches have been attempted to treat obese patients, it is widely recognized that the best long-term results are provided by bariatric surgery [20]. At present, three major surgical interventions are adopted to treat obese patients, i.e. sleeve gastrectomy, Roux-en-Y-gastric bypass, and laparoscopic adjustable gastric banding. Concerning the effects of this kind of surgery on gastrointestinal motility, it is worth noting that most studies report short (less than one year) follow-up periods. With respect to the influence of specific interventions on gut motility, only limited data are available. Sleeve gastrectomy tends to increase gastric emptying, Roux-en-Y-gastric bypass improves reflux symptoms and acid exposure, and laparoscopic adjustable gastric banding accelerates gastric emptying and affects esophageal motility [20].

Chronic intestinal pseudo-obstruction is a condition characterized by severe abnormalities of the propulsive activity of the gut, resembling mechanical obstruction. The therapeutic approach involves nutritional, pharmacological and surgical therapies, but the long-term outcome is poor in the vast majority of cases [21]. In this condition, surgery has a limited role, in that it may lead to disease progression and adhesion formation; of the various surgical options, only gastrostomies or jejunostomies may be useful for feeding, and defunctioning or venting gastrostomies or enterostomies may improve gastric/small bowel distension-related symptoms [22]. However, recent progress in small intestinal transplantation provides these patients with a better and more definitive alternative [23].

Colorectal Surgery

Sphincter-Preserving Surgery

Anterior resection of the rectum is carried out in a substantial number (up to 80%) of patients with colorectal cancer; most of these patients will subsequently develop a variety of bowel habit changes, including an increased number of evacuations, fecal incontinence, and abnormal evacuatory function [24]. This wide spectrum of motor disturbances, whose causes are still to be established, constitutes the so-called anterior resection syndrome [24]. Some pathophysiologic data may be summarized as follows [24]: (1) There is frequently a decrease in the basal resting pressure of the anal sphincter, a decrease that persists over time following resection. (2) Rectal capacity and compliance are impaired due to the surgical approach, resulting in a hypocompliant rectum whose reservoir function is totally or partially lost. Consequently, patients may experience bowel frequency, urgency, and fecal incontinence. Interestingly, it appears that the various reconstructive techniques following resection have a similar clinical outcome. (3) Colonic motility after anterior resection of the rectum has been evaluated in only very few studies, all demonstrating a major disturbance in colonic motor activity following surgery. Abnormalities have included an increase in the number of high-amplitude propagated colonic contractions that will contribute, together with the absence of the reservoir/braking function of the rectum, to the genesis of symptoms [25].

Of course, segmental resections will affect large bowel function depending on the resected segment. For instance, in the early postoperative period, left hemicolectomy has a major inhibitory effect on distal colonic motility, compared to nonanastomotic surgery of similar severity, whereas right hemicolectomy seems to modify only slightly colonic motor function, even in the long-term [26].

A surgical approach is sometimes needed for intractable constipation [27]. Concerning slow transit constipation, although the best results seem to rely on subtotal colectomy with ileorectal anastomosis, segmental resections are still carried out; as a consequence, greater or lesser lengths of diseased, frequently hypomotile colon, are left in situ, meaning that the likelihood of persisting problems is very high. Anyway, before referring a constipated patient for surgery, it is always wise to examine him/her quite extensively to exclude concomitant gut dysmotilities that could prejudice the outcome [27]. The surgical approach to obstructed defecation has, to date, largely relied on the stapled transanal rectal resection. While this approach is able to correct the anatomic abnormalities in about 50% of cases, the clinical outcome in the medium term is even less satisfying due to the profound modification of rectal compliance and the interference on pain perception that results in poor quality of life.

Rectopexy does not modify colonic motor variables in constipated patients with rectal prolapse [28]. Another surgical modality to treat refractory constipation, especially in children, is to perform an appendicostomy that allows large bowel irrigation; the few studies available concerning motility assessment in these circumstances have revealed a profound impairment of colonic motility in these subjects [27].

Hirschsprung's Disease

To date, a surgical approach is the only treatment available for these patients; however, it must be kept in mind that most of these patients will maintain an abnormal defecatory behavior after surgery [29]. The abnormalities consist of persistent constipation (related to an incomplete surgical resection or to abnormal colonic motility) or fecal incontinence (due to the damage to the internal anal sphincter caused by a lower level of dissection, vigorous anal dilation, and/or excessive anal canal traction during operation).

References

1 Bassotti G, Chistolini F, Sietchiping-Nzepa F, Morelli A: Intestinal manometry: value and limitations. Diabetes Nutr Metab 2004;17:33–37.

2 Bassotti G, Germani U, Morelli A: Human colonic motility: physiological aspects. Int J Colorectal Dis 1995;10:173–180.

3 Bassotti G, Germani U, Morelli A: Flatus-related colorectal and anal motor events. Dig Dis Sci 1996; 41:335–338.

4 Augestad KN, Delaney CP: Postoperative ileus: impact of pharmacologic treatment, laparoscopic surgery and enhanced recovery pathways. World J Gastroenterol 2010;16:2067–2074.

5 Doorly MG, Senagore AJ: Pathogenesis and clinical and economic consequences of postoperative ileus. Surg Clin North Am 2012;92:259–272.

6 van Bree SHW, Nemethova A, Cailotto C, Gomez-Pinilla PJ, Matteoli G, Boeckxstaens GE: New therapeutic strategies for postoperative ileus. Nat Rev Gastroenterol Hepatol 2012;9:675–683.

7 Bassotti G, D'Onofrio V, Battaglia E, Fiorella S, Dughera L, Iaquinto G, Mazzocchi A, Morelli A, Annese V: Treatment with botulinum toxin of octo-nonagerians with oesophageal achalasia: a two-year follow-up study. Aliment Pharmacol Ther 2006;23: 1615–1619.

8 Boeckxstaens GE, Annese V, des Varannes SB, Chaussade S, Costantini M, Cuttitta A, Elizalde JI, Fumagalli U, Gaudric M, Rohof WO, Smout AJ, Tack J, Zwinderman AH, Zaninotto G, Busch OR, European Achalasia Trial Investigators: Pneumatic dilation versus laparoscopic Heller's myotomy for idiopathic achalasia. N Engl J Med 2011;364:1807–1816.

9 Molena D, Yang SC: Surgical management of end-stage achalasia. Semin Thorac Cardiovasc Surg 2012; 24:19–26.

10 Hsu HS, Wang CY, Hsieh CC, Huang MH: Short-segment colon interposition for end-stage achalasia. Ann Thorac Surg 2003;76:1706–1710.

11 Bulsiewicz WJ, Madanick RD: Antireflux surgery in the proton pump inhibitor era. Cleve Clin J Med 2012;79:273–281.

12 Aprea G, Ferronetti A, Canfora A, Cardin F, Giugliano A, Guida F, Braun A, Battaglini Ciciriello M, Tovecci F, Mastrobuoni G, Amato B: GERD in elderly patients: surgical treatment with Nissen-Rossetti laparoscopic technique, outcome. BMC Surg 2012;12(suppl 1):S4.

13 Wilshire CL, Niebisch S, Watson TJ, Litle VR, Peyre CG, Jones CE, Peters JH: Dysphagia postfundoplication: more commonly hiatal outflow resistance than poor esophageal body motility. Surgery 2012;152: 584–592.

14 Pandolfino JE, Roman S: High-resolution manometry: an atlas of esophageal motility disorders and findings of GERD using esophageal pressure topography. Thorac Surg Clin 2011;21:465–475.
15 Nano M, Battaglia E, Gasparri G, Dughera L, Casalegno PA, Bellone G, Tibaudi D, Gramigni C, Ferronato M, Chiusa L, Navino M, Solej M, Dei Poli M, Emanuelli G: Decreased expression of stem cell factor in esophageal and gastric mucosa after esophagogastric anastomosis for cancer: potential relevance to motility. Ann Surg Oncol 2003;10:801–809.
16 Bassotti G, Gullà P, Betti C, Whitehead WE, Morelli A: Manometric evaluation of jejunal limb after total gastrectomy and Roux-Orr anastomosis for gastric cancer. Br J Surg 1990;77:1025–1029.
17 Bassotti G, Chiarinelli ML, Germani U, Chiarioni G, Morelli A: Effect of some abdominal surgical operations on small bowel motility in humans: our experience. J Clin Gastroenterol 1995;21:211–216.
18 El Halabi HM, Lawrence W Jr: Clinical results of various reconstructions employed after total gastrectomy. J Surg Oncol 2008;97:186–192.
19 Lee MS, Ahn SH, Lee JH, Park do J, Lee HJ, Kim HH, Yang HK, Kim N, Lee WW: What is the best reconstruction method after distal gastrectomy for gastric cancer? Surg Endosc 2012;26:1539–1547.
20 Ardila-Hani A, Soffer EE: Review article: the impact of bariatric surgery on gastrointestinal motility. Aliment Pharmacol Ther 2011;34:825–831.
21 Cogliandro RF, De Giorgio R, Barbara G, Cogliandro L, Concordia A, Corinaldesi R, Stanghellini V: Chronic intestinal pseudo-obstruction. Best Pract Res Clin Gastroenterol 2007;21:657–669.
22 Pakarinen MP, Kurvinen A, Koivusalo AI, Ruuska T, Mäkisalo H, Jalanko H, Rintala RJ: Surgical treatment and outcomes of severe pediatric intestinal motility disorders requiring parenteral nutrition. J Pediatr Surg 2013;48:333–338.
23 Millar AJ, Gupte G, Sharif K: Intestinal transplantation for motility disorders. Semin Pediatr Surg 2009;18:258–262.
24 Bryant CL, Lunniss P, Knowles CH, Thaha MA, Chan CLH: Anterior resection syndrome. Lancet Oncol 2012;13:e403–e408.
25 Bassotti G, de Roberto G, Chistolini F, Morelli A, Pucciani F: Case report: colonic manometry reveals abnormal propulsive behaviour after anterior resection of the rectum. Dig Liver Dis 2005;37:124–128.
26 Baxter NN, Pemberton JH: Postoperative motility disorders; in Schuster MM, Crowell MD, Koch KL (eds): Schuster Atlas of Gastrointestinal Motility, ed 2. Hamilton, BC Decker, 2002, pp 353–370.
27 Levitt MA, Mathis KL, Pemberton JH: Surgical treatment for constipation in children and adults. Best Pract Res Clin Gastroenterol 2011;25:167–179.
28 Brown AJ, Nicol L, Anderson JH, McKee RF, Finlay IG: Prospective study of the effect of rectopexy on colonic motility in patients with rectal prolapse. Br J Surg 2005;92:1417–1422.
29 Dasgupta R, Langer JC: Evaluation and management of persistent problems after surgery for Hirschsprung disease in a child. J Pediatr Gastroenterol Nutr 2008;46:13–19.

Prof. Gabrio Bassotti
Clinica di Gastroenterologia ed Epatologia, Ospedale Santa Maria della Misericordia
Piazzale Menghini, 1
IT–06156 San Sisto, Perugia (Italy)
E-Mail gabassot@tin.it

Author Index

Subject Index